It's easy to get lost in the cancer world

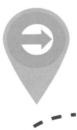

Let
NCCN Guidelines for Patients®
be your guide

✓ Step-by-step guides to the cancer care options likely to have the best results

✓ Based on treatment guidelines used by health care providers worldwide

✓ Designed to help you discuss cancer treatment with your doctors

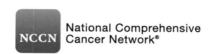

NCCN Guidelines for Patients® are developed by the National Comprehensive Cancer Network® (NCCN®)

NCCN

✓ An alliance of leading cancer centers across the United States devoted to patient care, research, and education

Cancer centers that are part of NCCN:
NCCN.org/cancercenters

NCCN Clinical Practice Guidelines in Oncology (NCCN Guidelines®)

✓ Developed by doctors from NCCN cancer centers using the latest research and years of experience

✓ For providers of cancer care all over the world

✓ Expert recommendations for cancer screening, diagnosis, and treatment

Free online at
NCCN.org/guidelines

NCCN Guidelines for Patients

✓ Present information from the NCCN Guidelines in an easy-to-learn format

✓ For people with cancer and those who support them

✓ Explain the cancer care options likely to have the best results

Free online at
NCCN.org/patientguidelines

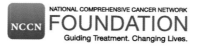
Guiding Treatment. Changing Lives.

and supported by funding from NCCN Foundation®

These NCCN Guidelines for Patients are based on the NCCN Guidelines® for Prostate Cancer (Version 2.2020, May 21, 2020).

NCCN Foundation seeks to support the millions of patients and their families affected by a cancer diagnosis by funding and distributing NCCN Guidelines for Patients. NCCN Foundation is also committed to advancing cancer treatment by funding the nation's promising doctors at the center of innovation in cancer research. For more details and the full library of patient and caregiver resources, visit NCCN.org/patients.

National Comprehensive Cancer Network (NCCN) / NCCN Foundation
3025 Chemical Road, Suite 100
Plymouth Meeting, PA 19462
215.690.0300

Endorsed by

California Prostate Cancer Coalition (CPCC)

CPCC is pleased to endorse this important resource. We believe it to be the most understandable and comprehensive guide for men diagnosed with prostate cancer who want to really understand what the disease is about and what their specific treatment options are. prostatecalif.org

Malecare Cancer Support

Malecare Cancer Support group members know that nothing is more perplexing than prostate cancer treatment choice making. The NCCN Patient Guidelines provide an excellent starting point for discussion, particularly for African Americans who die from prostate cancer at twice the rate as Caucasian men. malecare.org

National Alliance of State Prostate Cancer Coalitions (NASPCC)

NASPCC strongly endorses the NCCN Guidelines for Patients Prostate Cancer Advanced Stage, as an invaluable resource for patients and others. It is a reliable wealth of important information about prostate cancer in an understandable format. naspcc.org

National Prostate Cancer Awareness Foundation (PCaAware)

A wonderful resource for patients seeking a better and clearer understanding of the journey that lies ahead. pcaaware.org

Prostate Cancer Foundation

The Prostate Cancer Foundation is the world's leading philanthropic organization dedicated to funding life-saving cancer research. The NCCN Patient Guidelines Prostate Cancer Advanced Stage outlines essential information about diagnosis and treatment in a comprehensible format. They serve as a foundation of knowledge as patients and families begin to discuss treatment options with their health care provider. pcf.org

Urology Care Foundation

The Urology Care Foundation is the world's leading nonprofit urological health foundation – and the official foundation of the American Urological Association. As an organization that strongly believes in providing prostate cancer patients, caregivers, and those impacted by this disease the educational tools and resources necessary to make informed care and treatment decisions, we are pleased to endorse the NCCN Guidelines for Patients. urologyhealth.org

Veterans Prostate Cancer Awareness

Veterans Prostate Cancer Awareness commends the National Comprehensive Cancer Network (NCCN) for developing the Patient Guidelines for use as the standard in education and awareness for prostate cancer patients and providers. On behalf of all Veterans, VPCa thanks NCCN for providing this valuable tool to use as guidance on the journey through prostate cancer. vetsprostate.org

ZERO – The End of Prostate Cancer

Every 16 minutes a man loses his battle with prostate cancer. As the leading national prostate cancer advocacy organization, ZERO is proud to support NCCN Guidelines for Patients, a premiere resource to help patients and families navigate their prostate cancer journey. Additional free resources and support programs for the prostate cancer community can be found at zerocancer.org

With generous support from

Marianne and Donald Green

Francine Parnes

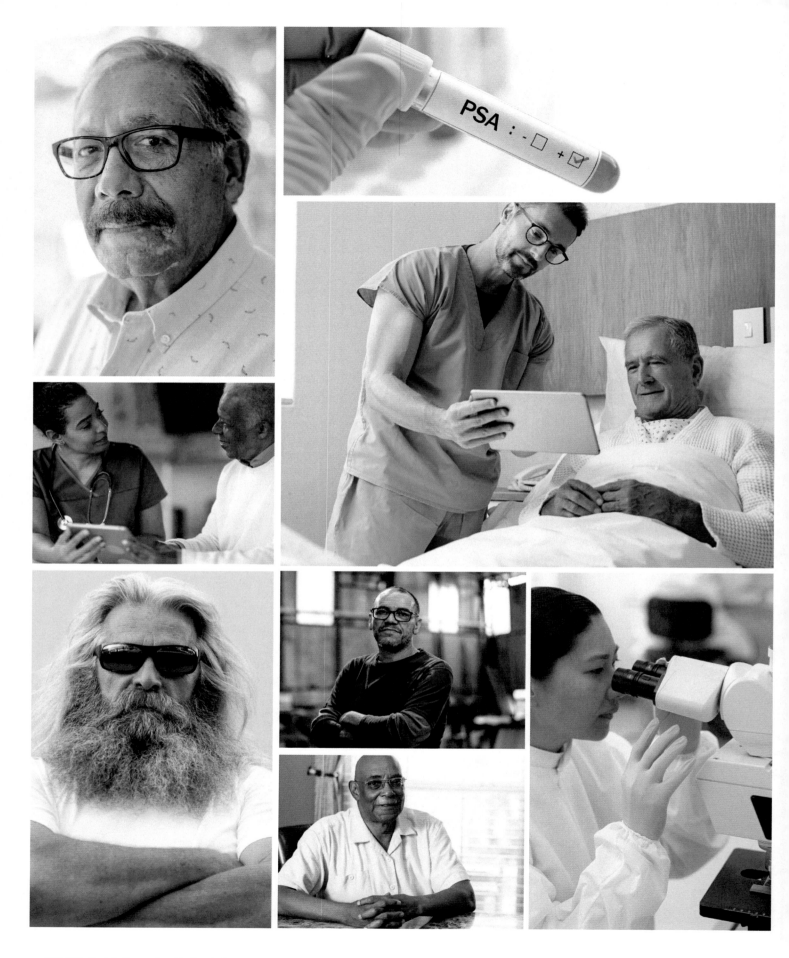

Contents

1
Prostate cancer basics

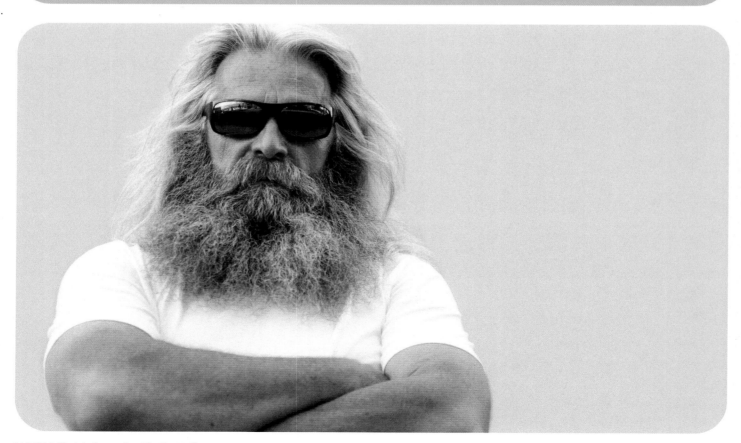

The prostate is a gland located below the bladder. In advanced prostate cancer, cancer cannot be cured with surgery or radiation therapy. Advanced prostate cancer can be metastatic, but not always. This chapter presents an overview of prostate cancer.

The prostate

The prostate is a walnut-sized gland. A gland is an organ that makes fluids or chemicals the body needs. The prostate gland produces a white-colored fluid that is part of semen. Semen is made up of sperm from the testicles and fluid from the prostate and other sex glands. During ejaculation, semen is released from the body through the penis.

The prostate is found below the bladder near the base of the penis and in front of the rectum. The prostate can be felt during a rectal exam. As a man ages, the prostate tends to grow larger.

The prostate surrounds the urethra. The urethra is a tube that carries urine from the bladder and out of the body. Above the prostate and behind the bladder are two seminal vesicles. Seminal vesicles are also glands that make a fluid that is part of semen. Semen leaves the body through the urethra.

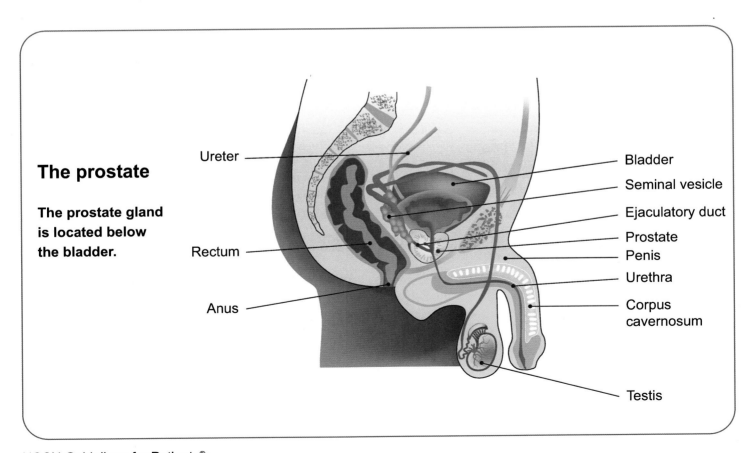

The prostate

The prostate gland is located below the bladder.

Ureter — Bladder
— Seminal vesicle
— Ejaculatory duct
— Prostate
Rectum — — Penis
— Urethra
Anus — — Corpus cavernosum
— Testis

Facts about prostate cancer

A risk factor is anything that increases your chance of cancer.

A few facts:

> - All men are at risk for prostate cancer.

> - 1 out of 9 men will develop prostate cancer.

> - Age is the most common risk factor. The older a man is, the greater the chance of getting prostate cancer.

African-American men

All men are at risk for prostate cancer, but African-American men are more likely to get prostate cancer and at a younger age. Cancer in African-American men tends to be more aggressive and more advanced. However, once diagnosed, African-Americans have similar treatment results as other men with the same cancer stage.

Family history

Men who have a family member with prostate cancer have a greater chance of getting prostate cancer. Those with a family history of certain cancers are at risk for prostate cancer.

How prostate cancer spreads

Cancer is a disease that starts in the cells of your body. Prostate cancer starts in the cells of the prostate gland. Almost all prostate cancers are adenocarcinomas. An adenocarcinoma is cancer in the cells that secrete fluids or other substances. Adenocarcinomas of the prostate are the focus of this book.

Unlike normal cells, cancer cells can grow or spread to form tumors in other parts of the body.

Cancer that has spread is called a metastasis.

> - Cancer that is contained entirely within the prostate is called **localized prostate cancer**.

> - Cancer that has spread from the prostate gland to nearby lymph nodes, but no further, is called **regional prostate cancer**.

> - Cancer that has spread beyond the prostate or regional lymph nodes is called distant metastasis, and may be referred to as **metastatic prostate cancer**.

Cancer can spread to distant sites through blood. Prostate cancer can metastasize in the bones, lymph nodes, liver, lungs, and other organs.

Cancer can also spread through the lymphatic system. The lymphatic system contains a clear fluid called lymph. Lymph gives cells water and food. It also has white blood cells that fight germs. Lymph nodes filter lymph and remove the germs. Lymph travels throughout the body in vessels like blood does. Lymph vessels and nodes are found everywhere in the body.

About this book

This book is for those with advanced prostate cancer or metastatic prostate cancer.

Advanced prostate cancer is cancer that cannot be cured with surgery or radiation. Advanced prostate cancer can be metastatic, but not always. For example, advanced cancers such as castration-resistant prostate cancer may or may not be metastatic.

Treatment for regional prostate cancer can be found at *NCCN Guidelines for Patients: Prostate Cancer, Early Stage* at NCCN.org/patientguidelines

Review

> The prostate gland makes a fluid that is part of semen.

> Prostate cancer starts in the cells of the prostate gland.

> Cancer cells can spread to other body parts through blood or lymph.

> All men are at risk for prostate cancer, but African-American men are more likely to get prostate cancer.

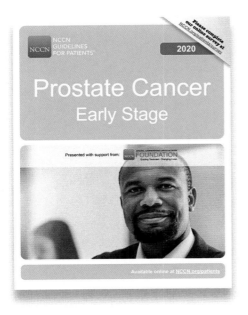

2
Prostate cancer tests

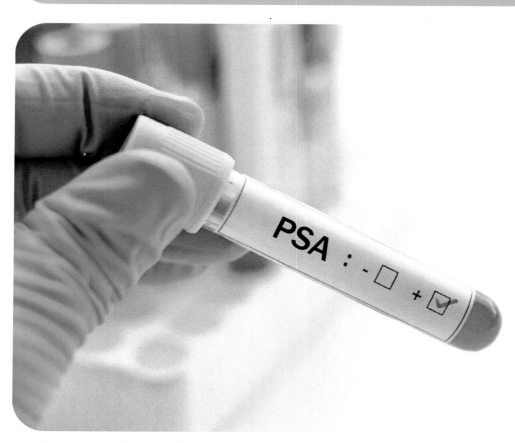

Testing is used to find and treat prostate cancer. A biopsy is needed to confirm cancer. This chapter presents an overview of tests you might receive and what to expect.

Test results

Results from blood tests, imaging studies, and biopsy will be used to determine your treatment plan. It is important you understand what these tests mean. Ask questions and keep copies of your test results. Online patient portals are a great way to access your test results.

Whether you are going for a second opinion, test, or office visit, keep these things in mind:

> Bring someone with you to doctor visits, if possible.

> Write down questions and take notes during appointments. Don't be afraid to ask your care team questions. Get to know your care team and let them get to know you.

> Get copies of blood tests, imaging results, and reports about the specific type of cancer you have.

> Organize your papers. Create files for insurance forms, medical records, and test results. You can do the same on your computer.

> Keep a list of contact information for everyone on your care team. Add it to your binder or notebook. Hang the list on your fridge or keep it by the phone.

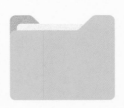

Create a medical binder

A medical binder or notebook is a great way to organize all of your records in one place.

- Make copies of blood tests, imaging results, and reports about your specific type of cancer. It will be helpful when getting a second opinion.

- Choose a binder that meets your needs. Consider a zipper pocket to include a pen, small calendar, and insurance cards.

- Create folders for insurance forms, medical records, and tests results. You can do the same on your computer.

- Use online patient portals to view your test results and other records. Download or print the records to add to your binder.

- Organize your binder in a way that works for you. Add a section for questions and to take notes.

- Bring your medical binder to appointments. You never know when you might need it!

General health tests

Medical history

A medical history is a record of all health issues and treatments you have had in your life. Be prepared to list any illness or injury and when it happened. Bring a list of old and new medicines and any over-the-counter medicines, herbals, or supplements you take. Tell your doctor about any symptoms you have. A medical history will help determine which treatment is best for you.

Family history

Some cancers and other diseases can run in families. Your doctor will ask about the health history of family members who are blood relatives. This information is called a family history. It is important to ask members from both your mother's and father's side of the family about all cancers, not just prostate cancer. Ask about other health issues like heart disease and diabetes, at what age they were diagnosed, and if anyone died from their cancer. Share this information and any changes to family history with your health care provider.

Physical exam

During a physical exam, a doctor will check your body for signs of disease.

A health care provider will:

> Check your temperature, blood pressure, pulse, and breathing rate

> Weigh you

> Listen to your lungs and heart

> Look in your eyes, ears, nose, and throat

> Feel and apply pressure to parts of your body to see if organs are of normal size, are soft or hard, or cause pain when touched. Tell your doctor if you feel pain.

> Feel for enlarged lymph nodes in your neck, underarm, and groin. Tell the doctor if you have felt any lumps or have any pain.

> Perform a digital rectal (prostate) exam to check your prostate.

Imaging tests

Imaging tests take pictures of the inside of your body. These tests are used to detect and treat prostate cancer. Imaging tests show the primary tumor, or where the cancer started, and look for cancer in other parts of the body.

A radiologist, an expert who reviews test images, will write a report and send this report to your doctor. Your doctor will discuss the results with you. Feel free to ask as many questions as you like.

CT scan

A computed tomography (CT or CAT) scan uses x-rays and computer technology to take pictures of the inside of the body. It takes many x-rays of the same body part from different angles. All the images are combined to make one detailed picture.

A CT scan of your chest, abdomen, and/or pelvis may be one of the tests used to look for cancer that has spread to other areas (metastasized). CT scans are good at seeing lymph nodes and the area around the prostate.

Before the CT scan, you may be given contrast. Contrast materials are not dyes, but substances that help certain areas in the body stand out. Contrast is used to make the pictures clearer. The contrast is not permanent and will leave the body in your urine.

Tell your doctors if you have had bad reactions to contrast in the past. This is important. You might be given medicines, such as Benadryl® and prednisone, for an allergy to contrast. Contrast might not be used if you have a serious allergy or if your kidneys aren't working well.

MRI scan

A magnetic resonance imaging (MRI) scan uses radio waves and powerful magnets to take pictures of the inside of the body. It does not use x-rays. Like a CT scan, a contrast material may be used to make the pictures clearer.

An MRI might be used to look for prostate cancer that has metastasized to nearby lymph nodes in your pelvis.

mpMRI

A multiparametric MRI (mpMRI) is a special type of MRI scan. In an mpMRI, multiple scans are performed without contrast followed by another MRI with contrast.

You might have more than one mpMRI during the course of treatment. It might be done to learn more about your prostate cancer or to look for bleeding after a biopsy. An mpMRI might help detect certain types of tumors.

PET scan

A positron emission tomography (PET) scan uses a radioactive drug called a tracer. A tracer is a substance injected into a vein. Cancer cells show up as bright spots on PET scans. Not all bright spots are cancer. It is normal for the brain, heart, kidneys, and bladder to be bright on PET.

Often, a PET scan is combined with CT or MRI. This combined test is called a PET/CT or PET/MRI scan. It may be used to look for small tumors (metastases) in soft tissue and in bone.

Bone scan

A bone scan uses a radiotracer to make pictures of the inside of bones. A radiotracer is a substance that releases small amounts of radiation. Before the pictures are taken, the tracer will be injected into your vein. It can take a few hours for the tracer to enter your bones.

A special camera will take pictures of the tracer in your bones. Areas of bone damage use more radiotracer than healthy bone and show up as bright spots on the pictures. Bone damage can be caused by cancer, cancer treatment, or other health problems.

This test may be used if you have bone pain, are at high risk for bone metastases, or if there are changes in certain test results. Bone scans might be used to monitor treatment.

TRUS

A TRUS is a transrectal ultrasound. In this procedure, a probe is inserted into the rectum where high-energy sound waves are bounced off internal tissues to form an image called a sonogram. A TRUS is used to look for tumors in the prostate and nearby areas. A TRUS is also used to guide biopsies.

Blood tests

Blood tests check for signs of disease, how well organs are working, and treatment results.

Complete blood count

A complete blood count (CBC) measures the number of red blood cells, white blood cells, and platelets in your blood. Red blood cells carry oxygen throughout your body, white blood cells fight infection, and platelets control bleeding.

Blood chemistry

A blood chemistry test is another common type of blood test. This test measures the levels of different chemicals in the blood. Cancer or other diseases can cause levels that are too low or too high.

PSA

A prostate-specific antigen (PSA) measures a protein made by the fluid-making cells that line the small glands inside the prostate. These cells are where most prostate cancers start. You will have this test often.

Tissue tests

A biopsy is a procedure that removes samples of fluid or tissue. It is needed to confirm (diagnose) prostate cancer. Prostate cancer treatment often begins after biopsy.

A core biopsy or a core needle biopsy is the most common type of prostate biopsy. A hollow needle is used to remove one or more samples. Core samples will be taken from different parts of your prostate.

Biopsy samples will be sent to a pathologist. A pathologist is an expert who will test the biopsy and write a report called a pathology report. The pathologist may perform other tests to see if the cancer cells have specific genes or proteins. This information will help choose the best treatment plan for your type of cancer.

Genetic tests

Genes are coded instructions for the proteins your cells make. A mutation is when something is different in your genes than from most other people. Mutations can be passed down in families or can occur spontaneously. In other words, they may be present before you are born (inherited) or arise by genetic damage later in life (acquired).

Sometimes, genes inherited from your parents can increase the risk of different cancers. Depending on your family history or other features of your cancer, your health care provider might refer you for genetic counseling and testing to know if you have an inherited cancer risk.

There are 2 types of genetic tests:

> Genetic testing for inherited cancer risk

> Biomarker testing for cancer treatment planning

Genetic testing

Genetic testing is done using blood or saliva (spitting into a cup). The goal is to look for germline (inherited) mutations. Some mutations can put you at risk for more than one type of cancer. You can pass these genes on to your children. Also, family members might carry these mutations.

Examples of germline mutations for prostate cancer include *BRCA1, BRCA2, ATM, CHEK2, PALB2, MLH1, MSH2, MSH6,* and *PMS2* (for Lynch syndrome). Germline mutations like *BRCA1* or *BRCA2* are related to other cancers such as breast, ovarian, pancreatic, colorectal, and melanoma skin cancer.

If a germline mutation is suspected, you should be recommended for genetic counseling and follow-up germline testing. A genetic counselor is an expert who has special training in genetic diseases.

Germline testing is recommended for those with prostate cancer and any of the following:

> High-risk, very-high-risk, regional, or metastatic prostate cancer regardless of family history

> Ashkenazi Jewish ancestry

> A family history of high-risk germline mutations such as *BRCA1, BRCA2,* or Lynch syndrome mutation

> A strong family history of prostate cancer and certain other cancers

> Talk to your medical providers and/or a genetic counselor about your family history of cancer.

Biomarker testing

Biomarker (somatic) testing uses a sample from a biopsy of your tumor or cancer material to look for biomarkers or proteins. This information is used to choose the best treatment for you. Biomarker testing can be considered for those with localized, regional, or metastatic prostate cancer. Biomarker testing is sometimes called gene profiling or molecular testing.

HRRm

Your tumor might be tested for homologous recombination repair gene mutations (HRRm). These include *BRCA1, BRCA2, ATM, CHEK2, and PALB2.*

MSI testing

Microsatellites are short, repeated strings of DNA (the information inside genes). When errors or defects occur, they are fixed. Some cancers prevent these errors from being fixed. This is called microsatellite instability (MSI). Knowing this can help plan treatment. When cancer cells have more than a normal number of microsatellites, it is called MSI-H (microsatellite instability high). A next-generation sequencing (NGS) assay is the preferred MSI test.

MMR testing

Mismatch repair (MMR) helps fix mutations in certain genes. When MMR is lacking (dMMR), these mutations may lead to cancer. Knowing this can help plan treatment or predict how well treatment will work with your type of tumor.

Review

- › Tests are used to plan treatment and check how well treatment is working.

- › Online portals are a great way to access your test results.

- › Blood, imaging, and tissue tests check for signs of disease.

- › Imaging tests may be used to see if the cancer has spread beyond the prostate.

- › A biopsy is used to confirm (diagnose) prostate cancer.

- › A sample from a biopsy of your tumor might be tested to look for biomarkers or proteins.

- › Your health care provider might refer you for genetic counseling and testing to learn more about if you have inherited risk for cancer.

Bring a list of any medications, vitamins, over-the-counter drugs, herbals, or supplements you are taking.

3
Prostate cancer staging

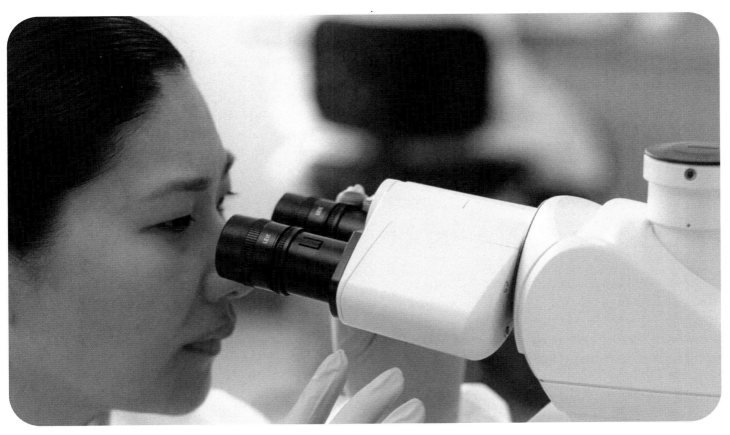

Cancer staging is how your doctors rate and describe the extent of cancer in your body. Doctors use cancer staging to plan which treatments are best for you.

Staging is based on a combination of factors listed below:

> - Digital rectal exam
> - PSA
> - Biopsy
> - Gleason score
> - Grade Group
> - TNM score

Digital rectal exam

A digital rectal exam is used to screen for cancer, rate the cancer stage, and assess how your cancer is responding to treatment. For this exam, your doctor will insert a lubricated, gloved finger into your rectum to feel your prostate for abnormalities. Not all parts of the prostate can be felt during this exam. It is more commonly called a prostate exam.

PSA

Prostate-specific antigen (PSA) is a protein made by the fluid-making cells that line the small glands inside the prostate. These cells are where most prostate cancers start. PSA turns semen that has clotted after ejaculation back into a liquid. Normal prostate cells, as well as prostate cancer cells, make PSA.

A small amount of PSA is made by all cells, even in women. PSA test results are one piece of information used for cancer staging, treatment planning, and checking treatment results.

PSA level
Serum PSA level is measured using a blood sample. PSA level is the number of nanograms of PSA per milliliter (ng/mL) of blood. Normal PSA levels vary by age and other conditions.

The larger the prostate, the more PSA it can make. Large prostates can be a result of cancer or other health issues. Some medicines, herbs, and supplements can also affect the PSA level. PSA increases after ejaculations and vigorous exercise, especially running or bicycling. Therefore, your doctor may recommend you refrain from sex and exercise before a PSA test. This will allow the PSA test to be more exact.

PSA density
PSA density (PSAD) is the amount of PSA compared to the size of the prostate. It is calculated by dividing the PSA level by the size of the prostate. The size of the prostate is measured by digital rectal exam, ultrasound, or an MRI scan.

PSA recurrence
When PSA levels rise after prostate cancer treatment with surgery or radiation therapy, it is called PSA recurrence. This could mean that the cancer has returned (recurrence) or that the treatment did not succeed in reducing the amount of cancer in the body (persistence).

PSA velocity and PSA doubling time

PSA velocity measures how fast PSA levels change over a period of time. How quickly this level increases could be a sign of prostate cancer and may help find a fast-growing prostate cancer. PSA doubling time (PSADT) is the time it takes for the PSA level to double.

Prostate biopsy

A biopsy removes a sample of tissue for testing. Rising PSA levels and an abnormal digital rectal exam may suggest cancer is present. However, the only way to know if you have prostate cancer is to remove tissue from your body and have a pathologist look at it under a microscope.

Types of biopsies

There are different types of biopsies used for prostate cancer. It is common to have more than one biopsy. A biopsy can be guided with an ultrasound, an MRI, or both.

Core biopsy

A core biopsy or a core needle biopsy uses a hollow needle to remove a tissue sample. Core samples will be taken from different parts of your prostate.

Transperineal biopsy

In a transperineal biopsy, a needle is placed into the prostate through the skin behind the testicles, an area known as the perineum.

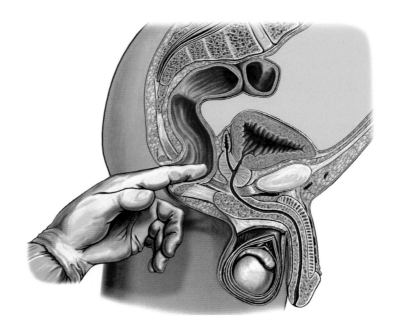

Digital rectal exam

Your prostate can be felt through the wall of your rectum. A digital rectal exam is a procedure during which your doctor will insert a finger into your rectum to feel your prostate.

Illustration Copyright © 2019 Nucleus Medical Media, All rights reserved. www.nucleusinc.com

TRUS-guided biopsy

A transrectal ultrasound (TRUS)-guided biopsy is the most common type of prostate biopsy. A sample of tissue is removed using a hollow needle that is inserted through the rectum (transrectal) and into the prostate. To ensure the best samples are removed, a TRUS is used to guide the needle. The TRUS uses sound waves to make a picture of your prostate that is seen by your doctor on a screen.

A spring-loaded needle will be inserted through the TRUS. Your doctor will trigger the needle to go through the rectal wall and into your prostate. The needle will remove tissue about the length of a dime and the width of a toothpick. At least 12 samples—called cores—are often taken. This is done to check for cancer in different areas of the prostate. Prostate biopsies aren't perfect tests. They sometimes miss cancer.

MRI-US fusion biopsy

An MRI-US fusion biopsy uses both an MRI and ultrasound. These images are then combined to help guide the biopsy. This will allow for better tracking of the movement of your prostate. It will also help doctors pinpoint which area of tissue to sample.

Prostate bed biopsy

After surgery to remove your prostate, a biopsy might be done of the area to look for signs that prostate cancer has returned or spread. This is called a prostate bed biopsy and might be done after PSA or imaging tests suggest cancer recurrence.

Metastatic lesion biopsy

Sometimes, a sample of a metastasis or metastatic lesion is taken for tumor testing. This helps to ensure that you will receive the best treatment for your type of cancer.

Prostate biopsy

There are different types of biopsies used for prostate cancer. It is common to have more than one biopsy. This image is of a transperineal biopsy.

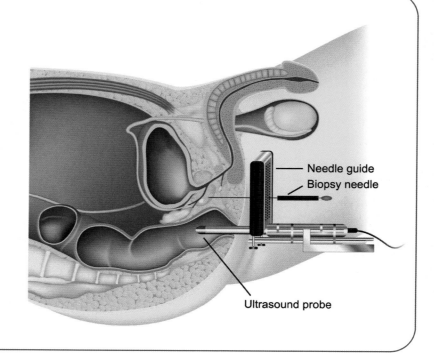

Needle guide
Biopsy needle
Ultrasound probe

Gleason score

The Gleason score describes how aggressive a prostate cancer is. A pathologist assigns this score after studying your biopsy under a microscope. It can be helpful to have a second pathologist review your biopsy to be sure the Gleason score is the same. The Gleason score is just one factor used by doctors to plan treatment.

A Gleason score is made up of two grades. A Gleason grade ranges from 1 to 5. A low grade of 1 means the cancer cells in your biopsy look very much like normal, healthy tissue. This is called well-differentiated. Cells that look very abnormal under a microscope are called poorly differentiated or undifferentiated, and have a grade of 4 or 5. The higher the grade, the more abnormal the biopsy looks and the more aggressive the cancer is. Most prostate cancers are grade 3 or higher.

Prostate tumors are given two grades. A primary grade is given to describe the cancer cells in the largest area of the tumor. A secondary grade is given to describe cancer cells in the second largest area of the tumor. When these grades are added together, it is called a Gleason score. For example, 3+4= a Gleason score of 7.

Gleason scores range from 2 to 10, but most prostate cancers are scored from 6 to 10. A Gleason score in the 8 to 10 range means the cancer is more likely to grow and spread quickly than a lower grade cancer. See Guide 1.

Guide 1 **Gleason score summary**	
6 or less	• The cancer is likely to grow and spread very slowly. • If the cancer is small, many years may pass before it becomes a problem. You may never need cancer treatment. • Also called **low grade.**
7	• The cancer is likely to grow and spread at a modest pace. • If the cancer is small, several years may pass before it becomes a problem. To prevent problems, treatment may be needed. • Also called **intermediate grade.**
8, 9, or 10	• The cancer is likely to grow and spread fast. • If the cancer is small, a few years may pass before the cancer becomes a problem. To prevent problems, treatment is needed now. • Also called **high grade.**

Grade Groups

Gleason scores are organized into Grade Groups. Grade Groups are meant to be simpler and more accurate. This method helps prevent overtreatment for those with low-grade prostate cancer. A Grade Group is just one factor used by doctors to plan treatment.

There are 5 Grade Groups. Grade Group 2 and Grade Group 3 both have a Gleason score of 7. The difference is the cancer in Grade Group 3 is more serious. If you look at the first number in the Gleason pattern (4+3) in Grade Group 3, it is higher than in Grade Group 2 (3+4). Remember, the first number or primary grade is given to rate cancer in the largest area of the tumor. See Guide 2.

Guide 2 Grade Groups	
1	• Gleason score 6 or less • Gleason pattern 1+3, 2+3, 3+3
2	• Gleason score 7 • Gleason pattern 3+4
3	• Gleason score 7 • Gleason pattern 4+3
4	• Gleason score 8 • Gleason pattern 4+4, 3+5, 5+3
5	• Gleason score 9 or 10 • Gleason pattern 4+5, 5+4, 5+5

TNM score

The American Joint Committee on Cancer (AJCC) created a way to determine how much cancer is in your body and where it is located. This is called staging. Staging is needed to make treatment decisions.

The tumor, node, metastasis (TNM) system is used to stage prostate cancer. In this system, the letters T, N, and M describe different areas of cancer growth. Based on cancer test results, your doctor will assign a score or number to each letter. The higher the number, the larger the tumor or the more the cancer has spread. These scores will be combined to assign the cancer a stage. A TNM example might look like this: T2, N0, M0. See Guide 3.

> **T (tumor)** - Size of the main (primary) tumor and if it has grown outside the prostate

> **N (node)** - If cancer has spread to nearby lymph nodes

> **M (metastasis)** - If cancer has spread to distant parts of the body or metastasized

Guide 3
Prostate cancer stage by TNM score

Stage	Primary tumor (T)	Regional lymph nodes (N)	Distant metastasis (M)
Localized	**T1** Tumor cannot be felt during digital rectal exam and is not found on imaging tests, but cancer is present.	**N0** There is no cancer in nearby lymph nodes.	**M0** Cancer has not spread to other parts of the body.
	T2 Tumor is felt during digital rectal exam and is found only in the prostate.	**N0**	**M0**
	T3 Tumor has broken through outside layer of prostate. It may have grown into seminal vesicle(s).	**N0**	**M0**
	T4 Tumor has grown outside the prostate into nearby structures such as the bladder, rectum, pelvic muscles, and/or pelvic wall.	**N0**	**M0**
Regional	**Any T**	**N1** There is cancer (metastasis) in nearby lymph nodes.	**M0**
Metastatic	**Any T**	**Any N**	**M1** Cancer has spread to other parts of the body (metastasized).

T = Tumor

T1 tumors cannot be felt during a digital rectal exam and are not found on imaging tests, but cancer is present. Cancer might be found by chance during a biopsy or surgery for another health issue related to the prostate or bladder. This is called an incidental finding.

> **T1a** means that incidental cancer was found in **5 percent (5%) or less** of the removed tissue.

> **T1b** means that incidental cancer was found in **more than 5 percent (5%)** of the removed tissue.

> **T1c** tumors are found by needle biopsy in one or both sides of the prostate.

T2 tumors can be felt by your doctor during a digital rectal exam. They also may be seen on an imaging test. T2 scores are based on whether the cancer is in one or both sides of the prostate. T2 tumors are found only in the prostate gland.

> **T2a** tumors involve half or less of one side of the prostate.

> **T2b** tumors involve more than half of one side of the prostate, but not both sides.

> **T2c** tumors have grown into both sides of the prostate.

T3 tumors have broken through the outside layer of the prostate gland. They might have reached the connective tissue around the prostate or the neck of the bladder.

> **T3a** tumors have grown outside the prostate, but not into the seminal vesicle(s).

> **T3b** tumors have grown outside the prostate and into the seminal vesicle(s).

T4 tumors have grown outside the prostate into nearby structures such as the bladder, rectum, pelvic muscles, and/or pelvic wall.

N = Node

There are hundreds of lymph nodes throughout your body. They work as filters to help fight infection and remove harmful things from your body. Lymph nodes near the prostate include the hypogastric, obturator, internal and external iliac, and sacral lymph nodes. Your doctor might refer to lymph nodes in the pelvis as pelvic lymph nodes. Most often, prostate cancer spreads to the external iliac, internal iliac, or obturator nodes. Cancer that has spread to lymph nodes near the prostate is shown as N1.

M = Metastatic

Cancer that has spread to distant parts of the body is shown as M1. Prostate cancer tends to metastasize in the bones and can spread to the liver, lungs, distant lymph nodes, and other organs.

Prostate cancer stages

There are many ways to describe prostate cancer. This can be very confusing.

Localized prostate cancer

Localized prostate cancer is cancer that is found only in the prostate. It has not spread to lymph nodes or distant organs.

TNM staging for localized prostate cancer might be one of the following:

> - T1, N0, M0
> - T2, N0, M0
> - T3, N0, M0
> - T4, N0, M0

Locally advanced prostate cancer

Locally advanced is a term used by some doctors to describe prostate cancer that has spread to nearby lymph nodes or organs like the bladder or rectum. This term may not be used in the same way by all doctors. If your doctor uses this term to describe your cancer, ask what it means.

Regional prostate cancer

Regional means prostate cancer has spread to nearby lymph nodes (N1). Nearby lymph nodes include the hypogastric, obturator, internal and external iliac, and sacral lymph nodes. Most often, prostate cancer spreads to the external iliac, internal iliac, or obturator nodes.

TNM staging for regional prostate cancer is:

> - Any T, N1, M0

Advanced prostate cancer

Advanced prostate cancer is cancer that cannot be cured with surgery or radiation. Advanced prostate cancer can be metastatic, but not always. For example, biochemical recurrence refers to a state where PSA is rising and suggests cancer recurrence, but there is no visible cancer on scans.

Metastatic prostate cancer

Metastatic (M1) prostate cancer has spread to distant parts of the body.

TNM staging for metastatic prostate cancer is:

> - Any T, Any N, M1

Review

> - Cancer staging describes how much cancer is in the body and where it is located.

> - Prostate cancer staging is based on digital rectal exam, PSA, prostate biopsy, Gleason score, Grade Group, and TNM score.

> - Digital rectal exam, PSA, and a prostate biopsy help determine the size of a tumor.

> - The Gleason score describes how aggressive a prostate cancer is.

> - Gleason scores are organized into Grade Groups for more accurate treatment.

> - The tumor, node, metastasis (TNM) system is used to stage prostate cancer.

4
Planning your treatment

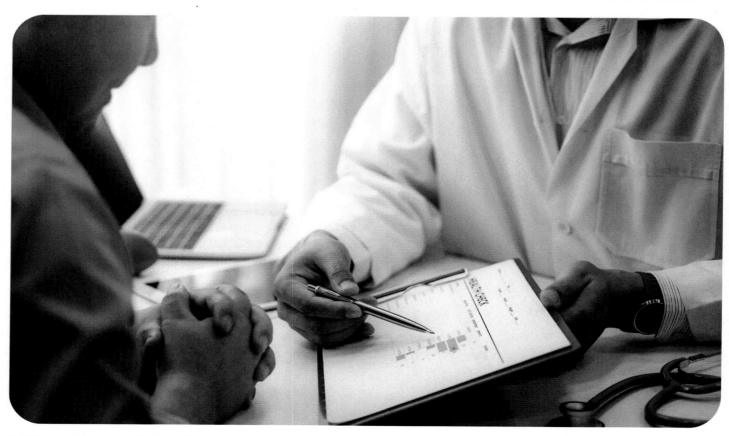

Many factors go into treatment planning. Your personal needs are important. This chapter discusses life expectancy, risk groups, and other factors that go into treatment planning.

Life expectancy

Life expectancy is the average life span of a person. It is measured in years. An estimate of your life expectancy is an important factor in deciding which tests and treatments you will need.

Prostate cancer often grows slowly. There may be no benefit to having tests or continuing treatment if you don't have any symptoms or if you have other more life-threatening health conditions.

Risk assessment

A risk assessment estimates the overall risk or chance that something will happen in the future. In the case of prostate cancer, a risk assessment will help to plan the best treatment for you. Before and during treatment, information will be collected about you and your cancer. Your risk assessment might change over time.

Your doctors will consider how likely the cancer:

> Might spread, how far, and how quickly

> Will respond to certain treatments

> Will return (called recurrence)

Doctors use these tools in risk assessment:

> Life expectancy

> Risk groups

> Nomograms

> Molecular testing (sometimes)

A risk assessment is not a guarantee. How your disease might progress is uncertain. You might do better or worse than your risk assessment.

Risk groups
Treatment options for prostate cancer are based on your risk group. The following information is used to determine your risk group:

> TNM score

> Gleason score and/or Grade Group

> PSA values

> Biopsy results

When you are first diagnosed, you will be placed into an initial risk group. See Guide 4.

Initial risk groups are:

> Very low

> Low

> Intermediate favorable

> Intermediate unfavorable

> High

> Very high

> Regional

> Metastatic

Guide 4
Initial risk groups

Very low

Has all of the following:
- T1c stage
- Grade Group 1
- PSA of less than 10 ng/mL
- Cancer in 1 to 2 biopsy cores with no more than half showing cancer
- PSA density of less than 0.15 ng/mL/g

Low

Has all of the following:
- T1 to T2a stage
- Grade Group 1
- PSA of less than 10 ng/mL

Intermediate

Has all of the following:
- No high-risk group features
- No very-high-risk group features
- 1 or more of the following intermediate risk factors:
  - T2b or T2c stage
  - Grade Group 2 or 3
  - PSA of 10 to 20 ng/mL

Favorable

Has all of the following:
- 1 intermediate risk factor
- Grade Group 1 or 2
- Less than half of biopsy cores show cancer

Unfavorable

Has one or more from below:
- 2 or more intermediate risk factors
- Grade Group 3
- More than half of biopsy cores show cancer

High

Has one from below:
- T3a stage
- Grade Group 4
- Grade Group 5
- PSA of more than 20 ng/mL

Very high

Has one from below:
- T3b to T4 stage
- Primary Gleason pattern 5
- More than 4 biopsy cores with Grade Group 4 or 5

Nomograms

A nomogram predicts the course your cancer will take, called a prognosis. It uses math to compare you and your prostate cancer to other men who have been treated for prostate cancer. Nomograms might be used to predict the extent of cancer and the long-term results for surgery or other treatment. A nomogram that predicts how likely prostate cancer has spread to your pelvic lymph nodes might be used when making treatment decisions. In addition to risk groups and other factors, nomograms are used to plan treatment.

Molecular tumor tests

Molecules are very tiny particles found in the cells of your body. There are special tests that measure certain molecules and biomarkers. A biomarker may be a molecule secreted by a tumor or a specific response in the body when cancer is present. When biomarkers are found, cancer may be present. PSA is an example of a biomarker used in detecting prostate cancer. This biomarker is found in a blood test.

Some molecular tests are done using prostate or lymph node tissue that was removed during biopsy. Results from these and other tests may help choose a treatment plan that is right for you.

If your doctor recommends molecular testing, it would be in addition to standard tests, such as PSA, Gleason grade, and imaging. You might have this test to see how well your body is responding to prostate cancer treatment. A molecular tumor test is also known as a molecular assay or analysis. If you have any questions about why you are having a test or what it means, ask your care team.

Metastases

Imaging tests can help show if the cancer has spread or metastasized in bones, lymph nodes, or other tissues. Treatment will depend on the type of metastasis.

There are different types of metastasis:

> Bone

> Lymph node and soft tissue

> Visceral (organ)

A bone scan is used to look for bone metastasis. Pelvic imaging with or without abdominal imaging is used to look for metastasis in the lymph nodes or other nearby visceral (internal) organs.

In prostate cancer, a visceral metastasis is cancer that has spread to the liver, lung, adrenal gland, brain, or an area inside the abdomen and pelvis. Lymph nodes are not considered visceral. You might have more tests if cancer is suspected in these or other areas of the body. Imaging tests to look for metastatic disease should not be performed if you are very low risk or low risk.

> Cancer that has metastasized in lymph nodes located near the prostate is called **regional prostate cancer**.

> Cancer that has spread to distant sites in the body is called **metastatic prostate cancer**.

Low-volume and high-volume are terms used to describe metastases.

> **Low-volume metastatic (M1) disease** includes lymph node metastases and/or 3 or fewer bone metastases.

> **High-volume metastatic (M1) disease** includes visceral metastases and/or 4 or more bone metastases with 1 or more bone metastasis outside the spine or pelvis.

If your life expectancy is more than 5 years or you have cancer symptoms, testing for metastases may help with treatment planning.

Get to know
your care team
and let them get
to know you.

Possible treatment side effects

A side effect is a problem or uncomfortable condition caused by treatment. Side effects are part of any treatment.

Possible side effects from prostate cancer treatment are:

> Urinary retention

> Urinary incontinence

> Erectile dysfunction

Often, these side effects are temporary and go away on their own. However, there is always a risk that a side effect may become long term or permanent. Talk with your doctor about your risk for these and other side effects, such as bowel problems, and how they might be prevented or treated.

Urinary retention
Urinary retention or the inability to completely empty the bladder. Your bladder might feel like it is full even after urinating.

Urinary incontinence
Urinary incontinence is the inability to control the flow of urine from the bladder. There are different degrees of incontinence.

Erectile dysfunction
Erectile dysfunction or impotence is the inability to achieve or maintain an erection. Erectile function after surgery will likely be close to what it was before surgery. But, it may be worse. Prostate surgery that spares the nerves near the prostate can help maintain erectile function and prevent urinary issues.

Treatment team

Treating prostate cancer takes a team approach. **It is important to see both a radiation oncologist and a urologist to discuss which treatment approach is right for you.**

Some members of your care team will be with you throughout cancer treatment, while others will only be there for parts of it. Get to know your care team and let them get to know you.

Depending on your diagnosis, your team might include the following:

> **Your primary care doctor** handles medical care not related to your cancer. This person can help you express your feelings about treatments to your cancer care team.

> **A pathologist** interprets tests on cells, tissues, and organs removed during a biopsy or surgery.

> **A diagnostic radiologist** reads the results of x-rays and other imaging tests.

> **An anesthesiologist** gives anesthesia, a medicine so you do not feel pain during surgery or procedures.

> **A urologist** is an expert in the male and female urinary tract and the male reproductive organs.

> **A urologic oncologist** specializes in diagnosing and treating cancers of the male and female urinary tract and the male reproductive organs.

> **An interventional radiologist** performs needle biopsies of tumors and ablative therapies.

> **A surgical oncologist** performs operations to remove cancer.

> **A radiation oncologist** prescribes and plans radiation therapy to treat cancer.

> **A medical oncologist** treats cancer in adults using systemic therapy, such as chemotherapy and hormone therapy. A medical oncologist will often coordinate your care. Ask who will coordinate your care.

> **Advanced practice providers** are an important part of any team. These are registered nurse practitioners and physician assistants who monitor your health and provide care.

> **Residents and fellows** are doctors who are continuing their training, some to become specialists in a certain field of medicine.

> **Oncology nurses** provide your hands-on care, like giving systemic therapy, managing your care, answering questions, and helping you cope with side effects.

> **Nutritionists** can provide guidance on what foods or diet are most suitable for your particular condition.

> **Psychologists and psychiatrists** are mental health experts who can help manage issues such as depression, anxiety, or other mental health conditions that can affect how you feel.

> **Genetic counselors** are experts who can help interpret how your family history may impact your treatment.

You know your body better than anyone. Help other team members understand:

> How you feel

> What you need

> What is working and what is not

Keep a list of names and contact information for each member of your team. This will make it easier for you and anyone involved in your care to know whom to contact with questions or concerns.

Review

> Doctors plan treatment using many sources of information.

> Life expectancy is the number of years you will likely live. It is used to plan treatment.

> A nomogram predicts the course your cancer will take, called a prognosis.

> A risk assessment is used to plan treatment. A risk assessment consists of life expectancy, risk groups, nomograms, and possible molecular tumor tests.

> You will be put into an initial risk group. This is based on your TNM score, Gleason score and/or Grade Group, PSA values, and biopsy results. Initial treatment will be based on your initial risk group.

> Side effects of prostate cancer may include urinary retention, urinary incontinence, and erectile dysfunction.

> Since surgery and radiation therapy have similar long-term cure rates, it is important to see both a radiation oncologist and a urologist to discuss which treatment approach is right for you.

5
Prostate cancer treatment

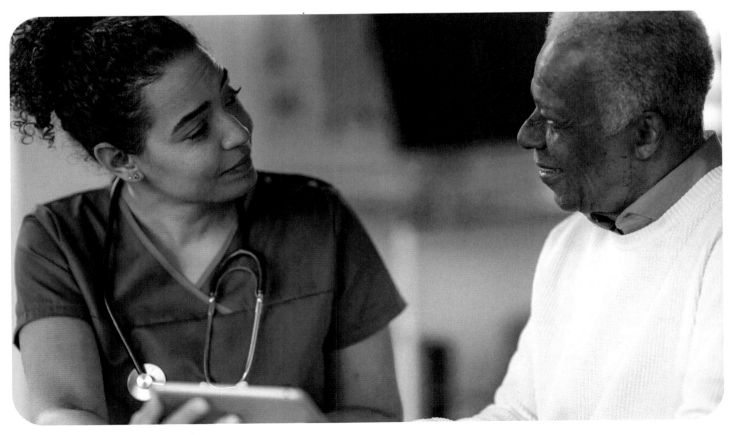

There is more than one treatment for prostate cancer. This chapter describes treatment options and what to expect. Discuss with your doctor which treatment might be best for you.

Prostate cancer is usually a slow-growing disease. It is a complex disease with many treatment options. Treatment can be local, systemic, or a combination of both. Local therapies target specific areas of the body that contain cancer cells. Systemic therapies attack cancer cells throughout the body.

There are 2 types of treatment:

> **Local therapy** focuses on a certain area. In prostate cancer, this treatment can include surgery, cryotherapy, radiation therapy, or high-intensity focused ultrasound (HIFU).

> **Systemic therapy** works throughout the body. It includes hormone therapy, chemotherapy, or other treatments designed to maintain or improve your quality of life.

Observation

Observation involves monitoring your prostate cancer and watching for symptoms. A rising PSA level or a change in a digital rectal exam might be a sign that you will soon have symptoms. The goal is to treat symptoms just before they are likely to start. This is so you have a good quality of life. Treatment is focused on palliation or symptom relief rather than curing the cancer.

Surgery

Surgery is a procedure to remove cancer from the body. The tumor will be removed along with some normal-looking prostate tissue around its edge called the surgical margin. A clear or negative margin (R0) is when no cancer cells are found in the tissue around the edge of the tumor. In a positive margin (R1), cancer cells are found in normal-looking tissue around the tumor. A negative margin (R0) is the best result.

Surgery can be used as the main or primary treatment. This may be only one part of a treatment plan. The type of surgery you receive depends on the size and location of the tumor. It also depends on whether there is cancer in any surrounding organs and tissues.

There are 2 types of surgery:

> Open surgery

> Minimally invasive surgery (laparoscopic or robotic surgery)

Open surgery
Open surgery removes the prostate through one large cut or incision. The large incision lets your doctor directly view and access the tumor to remove it.

Minimally invasive surgery
Minimally invasive surgery uses several small incisions or cuts instead of one large cut. Small tools are inserted through each incision to perform the surgery. One of the tools, called a laparoscope, is a long tube with a video camera at the end. The camera lets your doctor see your prostate and other tissues inside your body. Other tools are used to remove the tumor.

Radical prostatectomy

A radical prostatectomy is an operation that removes the entire prostate, seminal vesicles, and some nearby tissue. Pelvic lymph nodes may be removed.

A radical prostatectomy is often used when all of the following are true:

> The tumor is found only in the prostate

> The tumor can be removed completely with surgery

> You have a life expectancy of 10 or more years

> You have no other serious health conditions

A radical prostatectomy is complex and requires a great deal of skill. Surgeons who are experienced in this type of surgery often have better results.

After a radical prostatectomy, a catheter will be inserted into your urethra to allow your urethra to heal. It will stay in place for 1 to 2 weeks after surgery. You will be shown how to care for it while at home. If removed too early, you may lose control of your bladder (urinary incontinence) or be unable to urinate due to scar tissue.

A radical prostatectomy can be open or minimally invasive surgery. Staging before a radical prostatectomy is called **clinical (c) staging**. After a radical prostatectomy, your prostate will be tested to confirm cancer stage. This is called **pathologic (p) staging**.

There are 2 types of open radical prostatectomies:

> Retropubic

> Perineal

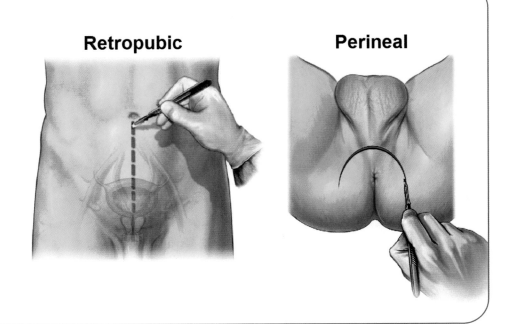

Open methods to radical prostatectomy

Your prostate may be removed through one large cut in your pelvis or between your legs.

Illustration Copyright © 2019 Nucleus Medical Media, All rights reserved. www.nucleusinc.com

Retropubic

Perineal

Radical retropubic prostatectomy

This surgery removes tissue through a cut that runs from your belly button down to the base of your penis. During the operation, you will lie on your back on a table with your legs slightly higher than your head.

Before removing your prostate, some veins and your urethra will be cut to clear the area. Your seminal vesicles will be removed along with your prostate. After removing your prostate, your urethra will be reattached to your bladder.

Your cavernous nerve bundles are on both sides of your prostate. These are needed for natural erections. A nerve-sparing prostatectomy will be done if your cavernous nerves are likely to be cancer-free. However, if cancer is suspected, then one or both bundles of nerves will be removed. If removed, good erections are still possible with the help of medication. You can still orgasm with or without these nerves.

Radical perineal prostatectomy

In a radical perineal prostatectomy a cut is made in your perineum. The perineum is the area between your scrotum and anus.

Your prostate and seminal vesicles will be removed after being separated from nearby tissues. An attempt will be made to spare nearby nerves. After your prostate has been removed, your urethra will be reattached to your bladder. Lymph nodes cannot be removed with this operation.

After surgery

Most men have temporary urinary incontinence and erectile dysfunction after a radical prostatectomy. These two side effects may be short lived, but for some men they are lifelong issues.

You're at higher risk for erectile dysfunction if 1) you're older, 2) you have erectile problems before surgery, or 3) your cavernous nerves are damaged or removed during surgery. If your cavernous nerves are removed, there is no good proof that nerve grafts will help restore your ability to have erections. Aids, such as medication, are still needed.

Removing your prostate and seminal vesicles will cause you to have dry orgasms. This means your semen will no longer contain sperm and you will be unable to have children.

Pelvic lymph node dissection

A pelvic lymph node dissection (PLND) is an operation to remove lymph nodes from your pelvis. It can be done as open retropubic, laparoscopic, or robotic surgery. PLND is usually part of a radical prostatectomy.

An extended PLND removes more lymph nodes than a limited PLND. An extended PLND is preferred. It finds metastases about two times as often as a limited PLND. It also stages cancer more completely and may cure some men with very tiny (microscopic) metastases.

Radiation therapy

Radiation therapy (RT) uses high-energy radiation from x-rays, gamma rays, and other sources to kill cancer cells and shrink tumors. Sometimes, it is given after surgery to reduce the chance that your cancer will return. Also, if your PSA begins to rise after surgery, RT might be recommended to try to kill the cancer cells that could have been left behind. It may be used as supportive care to help ease discomfort or pain in advanced and metastatic cancer.

There are 2 main types of radiation treatment:

> **External beam radiation therapy** (EBRT) uses a machine outside of the body to aim radiation at the tumor(s).

> **Internal radiation** is placed inside the body as a solid like seeds. This is called brachytherapy.

EBRT

There is more than one type EBRT used in the treatment of prostate cancer. These allow for safer, higher doses of radiation.

Types of EBRT that may be used to treat your cancer include:

> **Stereotactic body radiation therapy** (SBRT) uses high-energy radiation beams to treat cancers in five or fewer treatments.

> **Proton beam radiation therapy** uses streams of particles called protons to kill tumor cells.

> **Three-dimensional conformal radiation therapy** (3D-CRT) uses computer software and CT images to aim beams that match the shape of the tumor.

> **Intensity-modulated radiation therapy** (IMRT) uses small beams of different strengths to match the shape of the tumor. IMRT is a type of 3D-CRT that may be used for more aggressive prostate cancer.

> **Image-guided radiation therapy** (IGRT) uses a computer to create a picture of the tumor. This helps guide the radiation beam during treatment. IGRT is used with all of the types listed above to ensure that the radiation beams are always hitting the target. This spares normal tissues from radiation damage.

Brachytherapy

Brachytherapy is another standard radiation therapy option for prostate cancer. In this treatment radiation is placed inside or next to the tumor. Brachytherapy may be used alone or combined with EBRT, androgen deprivation therapy (ADT), or both. You might hear it called brachy (said braykey) for short.

Brachytherapy alone may be an option for men with very low-, low-, or favorable intermediate-risk prostate cancer depending on life expectancy. Those with high-risk cancers are not usually considered for brachytherapy alone.

There are 2 types of brachytherapy used to treat prostate cancer:

> Low dose-rate (LDR) brachytherapy

> High dose-rate (HDR) brachytherapy

LDR brachytherapy

Low dose-rate (LDR) brachytherapy uses thin, hollow needles to place radioactive seeds into your prostate. The seeds are about the size of a grain of rice. They are inserted into your body through the perineum and guided into your prostate with imaging tests.

The seeds usually consist of either radioactive iodine or palladium. They will stay in your prostate and give a low dose of radiation for a few months. The radiation travels a very short distance. This allows for a large amount of radiation within a small area while sparing nearby healthy tissue. Over time, the seeds will stop radiating, but will stay in your body (permanent).

HDR brachytherapy

High dose-rate (HDR) brachytherapy uses thin needles placed inside your prostate gland. These needles are then attached to tubes called catheters. Radiation will be delivered through these catheters. After treatment, the needles and catheters are removed.

Brachytherapy boost

Brachytherapy used with EBRT is called a brachytherapy boost, or brachy boost for short. LDR or HDR brachytherapy can be added as a boost to EBRT.

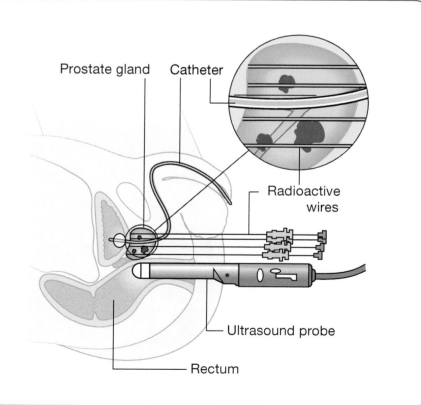

Brachytherapy

In brachytherapy, radiation is placed inside or next to the tumor.

https://commons.wikimedia.org/wiki/File:Diagram_showing_how_you_have_high_dose_brachytherapy_for_prostate_cancer_CRUK_419.svg

Prostate gland   Catheter

Radioactive wires

Ultrasound probe

Rectum

Systemic therapy

A cancer treatment that affects the whole body is called systemic therapy. It includes hormone therapy, chemotherapy, targeted therapy, and immunotherapy. Each works differently to shrink the tumor and prevent recurrence.

Ask your doctor about the goal of systemic therapy for your stage of prostate cancer. Be clear about your wishes for treatment. Systemic treatments may be used alone or together. See Guide 5.

Systemic therapies might include:

> **Chemotherapy** – attacks rapidly dividing cells in the body

> **Immunotherapy** – uses your body's natural defenses to find and destroy cancer cells

> **Biomarker-targeted therapy** – blocks the growth and spread of cancer by interfering with specific molecules

> **Bone-targeted therapy** - helps relieve bone pain or reduce the risk of bone problems

> **Hormone therapy** – adds, blocks, or removes hormones

Guide 5 Systemic therapies	
Chemotherapies	• Docetaxel • Mitoxantrone • Cabazitaxel • Cisplatin, carboplatin, and etoposide (only for small cell neuroendocrine prostate cancer)
Immunotherapies	• Sipuleucel-T
Biomarker-targeted therapies	• Rucaparib • Olaparib • Pembrolizumab
Bone-targeted therapies	• Denosumab • Zoledronic acid • Alendronate • Radium-223

*For horomone therapies, see Guide 6.

Immunotherapy

The immune system is the body's natural defense against infection and disease. It is a complex network of cells, tissues, and organs. The immune system includes many chemicals and proteins. These chemicals and proteins are made naturally in your body.

Immunotherapy is a type of systemic therapy that increases the activity of your immune system. By doing so, it improves your body's ability to find and destroy cancer cells. Immunotherapy is usually given alone when used for treating prostate cancer.

Sipuleucel-T

Sipuleucel-T (Provenge®) is a therapy that uses your white blood cells to destroy prostate cancer cells. Immune cells will be collected from your body and sent to a lab. Then, the immune cells will be activated or changed to target prostate cancer cells. This drug is known as a cancer vaccine.

Biomarker-directed therapy

In biomarker-directed therapy, treatment targets specific biomarkers such as programmed death receptor-1 (PD-1), *BRCA1/BRCA2*, and MSI-H/dMMR.

Examples of biomarker-targeted therapy include:

> Rucaparib (Rubraca™)

> Olaparib (Lynparza™)

> Pembrolizumab (Keytruda®)

Chemotherapy

Chemotherapy is a drug therapy that kills fast-growing cells throughout the body, including cancer cells and normal cells. All chemotherapy drugs affect the instructions (genes) that tell cancer cells how and when to grow and divide.

Chemotherapy drugs used to treat advanced prostate cancer include:

> Docetaxel

> Cabazitaxel

> Mitoxantrone hydrochloride

Docetaxel

Docetaxel (Taxotere®) is used to treat advanced prostate cancer. Docetaxel is an option for some men who are taking ADT for the first time. Docetaxel is also used to treat metastases after ADT fails to stop cancer growth.

Cabazitaxel

Cabazitaxel (Jevtana®) is an option if docetaxel doesn't work. However, the benefits of cabazitaxel are small and the side effects can be severe. You should not take cabazitaxel if your liver, kidneys, or bone marrow is not working well or if you have severe neuropathy, a nerve problem that causes pain, numbness, and tingling that starts in the hands and feet.

Mitoxantrone hydrochloride

Mitoxantrone hydrochloride (Novantrone® or DHAD) may relieve symptoms caused by advanced cancer.

Bone-targeted therapy

Medicines that target the bones may be given to help relieve bone pain or reduce the risk of bone problems. Some medicines work by slowing or stopping bone breakdown, while others help increase bone thickness.

When prostate cancer spreads to distant sites, it may metastasize in your bones. This puts your bones at risk for injury and disease. Such problems include bone loss (osteoporosis), fractures, bone pain, and squeezing (compression) of the spinal cord. Some treatments for prostate cancer, like hormone therapy, can cause bone loss, which put you at an increased risk for fractures.

There are 3 drugs used to prevent bone loss and fractures:

> Denosumab (Prolia®)

> Zoledronic acid (Zometa®)

> Alendronate (Fosamax®)

There are 3 drugs used to treat bone metastases:

> Radium-223

> Denosumab (Xgeva®)

> Zoledronic acid (Zometa®)

You will be screened for osteoporosis using a bone mineral density test. This measures how much calcium and other minerals are in your bones. It is also called a dual-energy x-ray absorptiometry (DEXA) scan and is painless. Bone mineral density tests look for osteoporosis and help predict your risk for bone fractures.

If you are at an increased risk for fracture, a baseline DEXA scan is recommended before starting hormone therapy. A follow-up DEXA scan after one year of hormone therapy is recommended.

Denosumab, zoledronic acid, and alendronate

Denosumab, zoledronic acid, and alendronate are used to prevent bone loss (osteoporosis) and fractures caused by hormone therapy. You might have blood tests to monitor kidney function and calcium levels. A calcium and vitamin D supplement will be recommended by your doctor.

Let your dentist know if you are taking any of these medicines. Also, ask your doctor how these medicines might affect your teeth and jaw. Osteonecrosis, or bone tissue death of the jaw, is a rare, but serious side effect. Tell your doctor about any planned trips to the dentist. It will be important to take care of your teeth and to see a dentist before starting treatment with any of these drugs.

Radiopharmaceuticals

Radiopharmaceuticals contain a radioactive substance that emits radiation. This radioactive substance is different than contrast material used in imaging.

Radium-223 collects in bone and gives off radiation that may kill cancer cells. The radiation doesn't travel far so healthy tissue is spared. Radium-223 is given though a vein (intravenous). You will have blood tests before each dose.

Since radium-223 leaves the body through the gut, common side effects are nausea, diarrhea, and vomiting.

Radium-223 is a radiopharmaceutical used to treat prostate cancer that has metastasized in the bone, but has not spread to other organs (visceral metastases). It is used in those whose prostate cancer is castration resistant. This is cancer that has not responded to treatments that lower testosterone levels (hormone therapy).

Radium-223 can be used with denosumab and zoledronic acid.

Hormone therapy

Hormone therapy is treatment that adds, blocks, or removes hormones. A hormone is a substance made by a gland in the body. Your blood carries hormones throughout your body.

The main male hormone or androgen is testosterone. Most of the testosterone in the body is made by the testicles, but the adrenal glands that sit above your kidneys also make a small amount.

Luteinizing hormone-releasing hormone (LHRH) and gonadotropin-releasing hormone (GnRH) are hormones made by a part of the brain called the hypothalamus. These hormones tell the testicles to make testosterone.

Hormones can cause prostate cancer to grow. Hormone therapy will stop your body from making testosterone or it will block what testosterone does in the body. This can slow tumor growth or shrink the tumor for a period of time. Hormone therapy can be local like in the surgical removal of the testicles (orchiectomy) or it can be systemic (drug therapy). The goal is to reduce the amount of testosterone in your body. See Guide 6.

Guide 6 Hormone therapies	
ADT	• Nilutamide, flutamide, or bicalutamide • Goserelin, histrelin, leuprolide, or triptorelin • Degarelix
Hormone therapy	• Enzalutamide, apalutamide, or darolutamide • Abiraterone with prednisone or methylprednisolone • Ketoconazole (may be used alone or with hydrocortisone) • Nilutamide, flutamide, or bicalutamide • Hydrocortisone, prednisone, or dexamethasone • DES or other estrogens
Surgery	• Orchiectomy

You might hear the term "castration" used when describing your prostate cancer or its treatment. This is the medical term for some types of hormone therapy. Castration can be temporary, a short-term treatment, or permanent like in an orchiectomy. If you are unsure what your doctor is talking about, ask.

Hormone therapy is not used by itself in the treatment of advanced prostate cancer.

There is one type of surgical hormone therapy:

> **Bilateral orchiectomy** is surgery to remove both testicles. Since the scrotum is not removed, implants might be an option.

The following are systemic (medical) hormone therapies:

> **LHRH agonists** are drugs used to stop the testicles from making testosterone. LHRH agonists include goserelin acetate, histrelin acetate, leuprolide acetate, and triptorelin pamoate. LHRH agonists will shrink your testicles over time.

> **LHRH antagonists** are drugs that block or stop the pituitary gland (attached to the hypothalamus) from making LHRH. This causes the testicles to stop making testosterone. Degarelix is an LHRH antagonist.

> **Anti-androgens** are drugs that block receptors on prostate cancer cells from receiving testosterone. Anti-androgens include bicalutamide, flutamide, nilutamide, enzalutamide, apalutamide, and darolutamide.

> **Estrogen** can stop the adrenal glands and other tissues from making testosterone. One type of synthetic estrogen made in a lab is called diethylstilbestrol (DES). Estrogen can increase the risk for breast growth and tenderness as well as blood clots.

> **Androgen synthesis inhibitors** are drugs that block androgen production. Ketoconazole is an antifungal drug that stops the adrenal glands and other tissues from making testosterone. Abiraterone acetate is similar to ketoconazole. Abiraterone is stronger and less toxic.

Androgen deprivation therapy

Androgen deprivation therapy (ADT) is treatment to suppress or block the amount of male sex hormones in the body. It is the primary or main systemic therapy for regional and advanced disease. ADT might be used alone or in combination with radiation therapy, chemotherapy, steroids, or other hormone therapies.

The term "hormone therapy" can be confusing. Some people refer to all hormone therapy as ADT. However, only orchiectomy, LHRH agonists, and LHRH antagonists are a form of ADT.

Palliative ADT

Palliative ADT is given to relieve (palliate) symptoms of prostate cancer. Palliative ADT can be given to those with a life expectancy of 5 years or less and who have high-risk, very-high-risk, regional, or metastatic prostate cancer. Palliative ADT can also be given to those who will start or have started to develop symptoms during observation.

Side effects of hormone therapy

Hormone therapy has side effects. Many factors play a role in your risk for side effects. Such factors include your age, your health before treatment, how long or often you have treatment, and so forth.

Side effects differ between the types of hormone therapy. In general, ADT may reduce your desire for sex and cause erectile dysfunction. If you will be on long-term ADT, your doctor may consider intermittent treatment to reduce side effects. Intermittent treatment is alternating periods of time when you are on and off ADT treatment. It can provide similar cancer control to continuous hormone therapy, but gives your body a break from treatment.

The longer you take ADT, the greater your risk for thinning and weakening bones (osteoporosis), bone fractures, weight gain, loss of muscle mass, diabetes, and heart disease. Other side effects of ADT include hot flashes, mood changes, fatigue, and breast tenderness and growth. Talk to your care team about how to manage the side effects of hormone therapy.

Calcium and vitamin D3 taken every day may help prevent or control osteoporosis for those on ADT.

Before ADT, you should receive a dual-energy x-ray absorptiometry (DEXA) scan to measure your bone density. Denosumab, zoledronic acid, or alendronate are recommended if your bone density is low. One year after treatment has started, another DEXA scan is recommended.

Diabetes and cardiovascular disease are common in older men. ADT increases the risk for these diseases. Thus, screening and treatment to reduce your risk for these diseases is advised. Tell your primary care physician if you are being treated with ADT.

ADT has been known to increase the risk of death from heart issues in African-American men. Ask your doctor about the risks of ADT treatment for your prostate cancer.

Corticosteroids

Corticosteroids or steroids are drugs created in a lab to act like hormones made by the adrenal glands. The adrenal glands are small structures found near the kidneys, which help regulate blood pressure and reduce inflammation (swelling). Corticosteroids stop the adrenal glands and other tissues from making testosterone. They are used alone or in combination with chemotherapy or hormone therapy.

Steroids to treat prostate cancer might include:

- Prednisone
- Methylprednisolone
- Hydrocortisone
- Dexamethasone

Thermal ablation

Thermal ablation uses extreme cold or extreme heat to destroy (ablate) cancer cells. It can destroy small tumors with little harm to nearby tissue. Cryosurgery and high-intensity focused ultrasound (HIFU) are two types of thermal ablation used to treat non-metastatic cancer that has returned (recurrence) after radiation therapy.

Cryotherapy

Cryotherapy is a procedure that damages prostate tumors through freezing. It is used to treat prostate cancer that has returned after radiation therapy. Cryotherapy is a treatment option if radiation therapy does not work.

Very thin needles will be inserted through your perineum into your prostate. The perineum is the space between your anus and scrotum. Imaging tests will be used to place the needles. Argon gas will flow through the needles and freeze your prostate to below-zero temperatures. Freezing kills the cancer cells. A catheter filled with warm liquid will be placed in your urethra to prevent damage to your urethra.

High-intensity focused ultrasound

High-intensity focused ultrasound (HIFU) uses high-energy sound waves that create heat to kill cancer cells. A probe is inserted into the rectum and the high-intensity sound waves are aimed directly at the cancer. HIFU (said high-foo) is a treatment option if radiation therapy does not work.

Clinical trials

A clinical trial is a type of research study that tests new methods of screening, prevention, diagnosis, or treatment of a disease.

Clinical trials have 4 phases.

> **Phase I trials** aim to find the safest and best dose of a new drug. Another aim is to find the best way to give the drug with the fewest side effects.

> **Phase II trials** assess if a drug works for a specific type of cancer.

> **Phase III trials** compare a new drug to a standard treatment.

> **Phase IV trials** evaluate a drug's long-term safety and effectiveness after it has been approved.

Those in a clinical trial often are alike in terms of their cancer type or stage and general health. This helps ensure that any change is a result of the treatment and not due to differences between participants.

If you decide to join a clinical trial, you will need to review and sign an informed consent form. This form describes the study in detail, including the risks and benefits. Even after you sign a consent form, you can stop taking part in a clinical trial at any time.

Ask your treatment team if there is an open clinical trial that you can join. Discuss the risks and benefits of joining a clinical trial with your care team. Together, decide if a clinical trial is right for you.

Review

> Observation looks for symptoms of cancer in order to treat the symptoms before they appear or get worse.

> Surgery removes the tumor along with some normal-looking tissue around its edge called a surgical margin. The goal of surgery is a negative margin (R0).

> A radical prostatectomy removes the prostate and the seminal vesicles. A pelvic lymph node dissection (PLND) removes lymph nodes near the prostate.

> Immunotherapy activates your body's disease-fighting system to destroy prostate cancer cells.

> Chemotherapy stops cancer cells from completing their life cycle so they can't increase in number.

> Hormone therapy treats prostate cancer by either stopping testosterone from being made or stopping what testosterone does in the body. It is the main systemic therapy for regional and advanced disease.

> Radiopharmaceuticals are radioactive drugs used to treat bone metastases.

> Radiation kills cancer cells or stops new cancer cells from being made.

> Cryotherapy kills cancer cells by freezing them and high-intensity focused ultrasound (HIFU) kills cancer cells by heating them.

> A clinical trial is a type of research that studies a treatment to see how safe it is and how well it works. Sometimes, a clinical trial is the preferred treatment option for prostate cancer.

Finding a clinical trial

Enrollment in a clinical trial is encouraged when it is the best option for you.

✓ To find clinical trials online at NCCN Member Institutions, go to **nccn.org/clinical_trials/ member_institutions.aspx**

✓ To search the National Institutes of Health (NIH) database for clinical trials in the United States and around the world, go to **ClinicalTrials.gov**

✓ To find clinical trials supported by the National Cancer Institute (NCI), go to **cancer.gov/about-cancer/treatment/ clinical-trials/search**

Ask your cancer team for help finding a clinical trial. You may also get help from NCI's Cancer Information Service (CIS). Call 1.800.4.CANCER (1.800.422.6237) or go to **cancer.gov/contact**

6
PSA persistence or recurrence

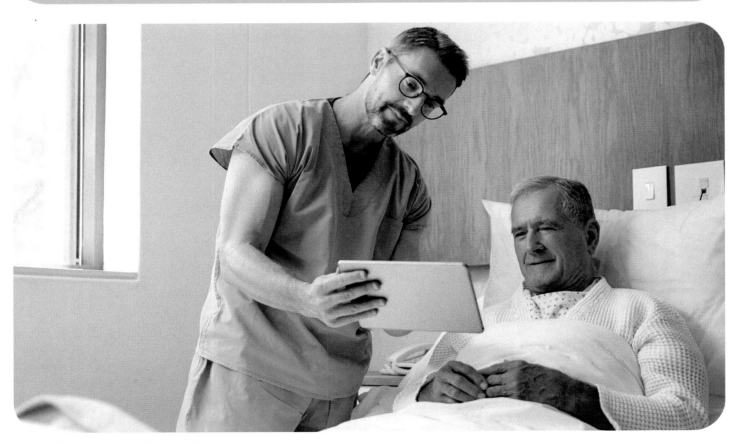

In PSA persistence, PSA levels do not lower after surgery or radiation therapy. When PSA levels fall to zero, but cancer later returns, it is called recurrence. PSA persistence or recurrence that happens after surgery is treated differently than PSA persistence or recurrence after radiation therapy.

PSA levels should be almost undetectable after a radical prostatectomy or external beam radiation therapy (EBRT). When PSA levels don't fall to near zero after treatment, it is called **PSA persistence**.

When cancer returns after PSA levels fall to near zero, it is called **recurrence**. Cancer may come back in the same place or in a different area of the body. Recurrence after a radical prostatectomy is treated differently than cancer that returns after EBRT.

Sometimes, cancer progresses to metastatic disease without PSA persistence or recurrence. This is called castration-naïve prostate cancer. Treatment for castration-naïve prostate cancer can be found in the next chapter.

After prostatectomy

Persistence
After a radical prostatectomy, your PSA level should fall to near zero since the whole prostate was removed. If this doesn't happen, it may be a sign of persistent cancer.

Recurrence
If your PSA level falls to zero or is undetectable, but later increases twice in a row, cancer may have returned (recurrence). The time it takes the PSA level to double will be calculated as PSA doubling time (PSADT).

Testing
Your doctor will consider the following tests:

- ➤ PSADT
- ➤ Bone scan
- ➤ Chest CT
- ➤ CT of abdomen and pelvis or MRI of abdomen and pelvis
- ➤ PET/CT or PET/MRI
- ➤ Prostate bed biopsy

Treatment

Treatment will be based on if tests find distant metastases. See Guide 7.

No metastases (M0)

If there are no distant metastases, then the treatment options are:

> EBRT

> EBRT with ADT

> Observation

Giving ADT with EBRT can prolong survival in certain patients. Intermittent ADT should be considered if you choose EBRT with ADT. If you are older and your PSADT is longer than 12 months, then observation is an option. Observation consists of testing on a regular basis so that palliative ADT can be given if symptoms from the cancer are likely to start.

ADT may include:

> LHRH agonist alone

> LHRH agonist with an anti-androgen

> LHRH antagonist

After treatment

After treatment, testing to monitor for disease progression will begin. If on ADT, testosterone levels will be measured.

Tests should include:

> Bone scan

> Chest CT

> CT of abdomen and pelvis or MRI of abdomen and pelvis

> PET/CT or PET/MRI (as needed)

Distant metastases (M1)

If distant metastases are found, then the treatment options are found under castration-naïve prostate cancer in the next chapter.

Guide 7
Treatment options: PSA persistence or recurrence after radical prostatectomy

No distant metastases	EBRT	
	EBRT with ADT	➡ When cancer progresses, See Chapter 7: castration-naïve prostate cancer
	Observation	
Distant metastases	See Chapter 7: castration-naïve prostate cancer	

After radiation therapy

After radiation therapy, PSA levels usually fall to near zero. If your PSA level falls to near zero, but later increases by at least 2 ng/mL, cancer may have returned. Other PSA changes might also be a sign of recurrence. Signs of cancer may be found in a digital rectal exam. The time it takes the PSA level to double will be calculated as PSA doubling time (PSADT).

A fast PSADT suggests cancer that has spread outside the prostate. It will be used to find your risk level. Imaging studies might be done to look for distant metastases.

Treatment

Treatment will be based on if you are a candidate for local therapy. Local therapy is treatment that focuses on the prostate. It includes radical prostatectomy with PLND, brachytherapy, cryotherapy, and high-intensity focused ultrasound (HIFU). Observation is also an option.

Local therapy is an option if all of the following are true:

> Original clinical stage was T1–T2, NX (cancer in lymph nodes can't be assessed) or N0

> Life expectancy of more than 10 years

> PSA is now at less than 10 ng/mL

For treatment options, see Guide 8.

Guide 8
Treatment options: PSA persistence or recurrence after radiation therapy

Local therapy is an option	TRUS biopsy finds cancer: • Observation • Radical prostatectomy with PLND • Brachytherapy • Cryotherapy • HIFU TRUS biopsy doesn't find cancer: • Observation • ADT	When cancer progresses, • See Chapter 7: castration-naïve prostate cancer • See Chapter 8: castration-resistant prostate cancer (CRPC)

To confirm that local therapy is right for you, tests will include:

> PSADT

> Bone scan

> Prostate MRI

> TRUS biopsy

Other tests might include:

> Chest CT

> CT of abdomen and pelvis or MRI of abdomen and pelvis

> PET/CT or PET/MRI

TRUS biopsy finds cancer

Local treatment options are based on if the TRUS biopsy finds cancer.

If TRUS biopsy shows cancer, the treatment options are:

> Observation

> Radical prostatectomy with PLND

> Brachytherapy

> Cryotherapy

> HIFU

TRUS biopsy does not find cancer

If TRUS biopsy does not find cancer, then treatment options are:

> Observation

> ADT

After treatment

After treatment you will be monitored for disease progression. If disease progression is suspected, then tests to confirm that cancer has grown or spread should include:

> Bone scan

> Chest CT

> CT of abdomen and pelvis or MRI of abdomen and pelvis

> PET/CT or PET/MRI (as needed)

Review

> When PSA levels rise after prostate cancer treatment with surgery or radiation therapy, it is called PSA recurrence. This could mean that the cancer has returned (recurrence) or that the treatment did not succeed in reducing the amount of cancer in the body (persistence).

> Cancer that returns after a radical prostatectomy will be treated differently than cancer that returns after radiation therapy.

> Persistence or recurrence after a radical prostatectomy is based on whether there are distant metastases.

> Persistence or recurrence after radiaton therapy is based on if local therapy is an option. Local therapy is treatment that focuses on the prostate.

7
Castration-naïve prostate cancer

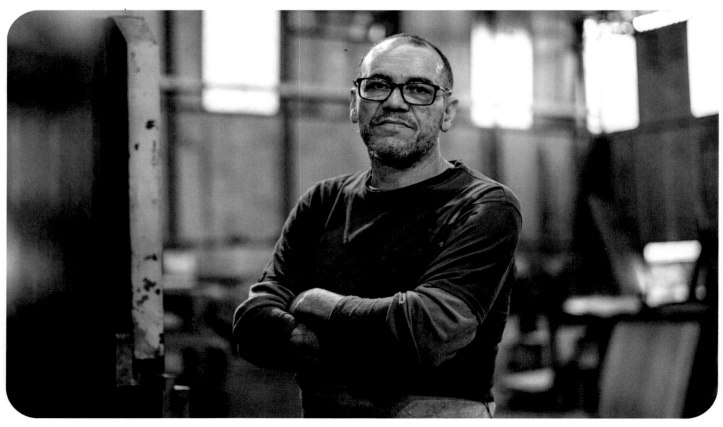

If you are not taking ADT and your prostate cancer progresses or gets worse, it is called castration-naïve prostate cancer. You can have castration-naïve prostate cancer if your initial or first diagnosis was metastatic prostate cancer.

Castration-naïve prostate cancer is usually treated with hormone therapy. This helps to prevent the spread of cancer. Treatment options for castration-naïve prostate cancer are based on if the cancer has metastasized (M1) or hasn't metastasized (M0). See Guide 9.

No metastases (M0)

If there are no metastases, the options are observation (preferred) or ADT.

Observation

Observation is the preferred option for castration-naïve prostate cancer without metastases (M0). Observation consists of testing on a regular basis so that palliative care with ADT can be given if symptoms from the cancer are likely to start. Tests during observation include PSA and digital rectal exam.

Hormone therapy

Surgical castration that removes both testes is called a bilateral orchiectomy. This surgery is a type of androgen deprivation therapy (ADT). An orchiectomy can be combined with other ADTs. Hormones such as an LHRH agonist or LHRH antagonist, or LHRH agonist with an anti-androgen are types of ADT used to treat this cancer.

ADT can be toxic and cause side effects. To reduce side effects, intermittent ADT might be

---

Guide 9
Treatment options: Castration-naïve prostate cancer

M0	• Observation (preferred) • ADT	→	Treatment followed by: • Physical exam with PSA every 3 to 6 months • Imaging for symptoms or increasing PSA
M1	ADT alone or with one of the following: • Apalutamide (preferred) • Abiraterone (preferred) • Docetaxel (preferred) • Enzalutamide (preferred) • Fine-particle abiraterone • EBRT to the primary tumor for low-volume metastases	→	Treatment followed by: • Physical exam with PSA every 3 to 6 months • Imaging for symptoms or increasing PSA

an option. Intermittent treatment alternates between periods of time when you are on and off ADT. It can provide similar cancer control to continuous hormone therapy, but gives your body a break from treatment.

Intermittent ADT often begins with continuous treatment that is stopped after about 1 year. Treatment is resumed when a certain PSA level is reached or symptoms appear. PSA levels that trigger restarting treatment may depend on rate of rise, time off therapy, PSA level at prior treatment, or other factors specific to the person. Intermittent ADT requires close monitoring of PSA and testosterone levels, especially during off-treatment periods.

LHRH agonists can cause an increase in testosterone for several weeks. This increase is called a "flare." Flare can cause pain if bone metastases can be seen on imaging tests (overt metastases). The pain doesn't mean the cancer is growing. You might be given a medicine to prevent flare.

Ask your doctor if you have concerns about the side effects of the ADT you are being prescribed and what might be done to prevent these side effects.

Metastases (M1)

You will have tests to confirm metastases.

Tests might include:

> Bone scan

> Chest CT

> CT of abdomen/pelvis or MRI of abdomen/pelvis with or without contrast

> PET/CT or PET/MRI

> Biomarker testing and genetic testing for inherited cancer risk

Treatment options will be ADT alone or with one of the following:

> Apalutamide (preferred)

> Abiraterone (preferred)

> Docetaxel (preferred)

> Enzalutamide (preferred)

> Fine-particle abiraterone

> EBRT to the primary tumor for low-volume metastases

Radiation therapy
EBRT might be added to ADT to treat bone metastases or for symptoms caused by prostate cancer.

Hormone therapy
An orchiectomy is a type of ADT. It can be combined with a chemotherapy or another hormone therapy. Drug forms of ADT are used alone or in combination with chemotherapy and other hormone therapies.

Monitoring

While on hormone therapy, your doctor will monitor treatment results. A rising PSA level suggests the cancer is growing. This increase is called a biochemical relapse. If PSA levels are rising, your testosterone levels should be tested to see if they are at castrate levels (less than 50 ng/dL). Castrate levels must be maintained.

Tests to monitor for disease progression include:

> Physical exam with PSA every 3 to 6 months

> Imaging for symptoms or increasing PSA

If the above tests show that your cancer might be growing or spreading, then the following tests are recommended:

> Bone scan

> Chest CT

> CT of abdomen with pelvis or MRI of abdomen with pelvis

> Consider PET/CT or PET/MRI

Disease progression

If your castration-naïve prostate cancer is getting worse, by growing or spreading and not responding to treatment, then it might be castration-resistant prostate cancer. This is discussed in the next chapter.

Review

> Cancer that progresses when you are not on androgen deprivation therapy (ADT) is called castration-naïve prostate cancer. It can be metastatic (M1) or non-metastatic (M0).

> M1 castration-naïve prostate cancer is treated with ADT alone or with another therapy like EBRT, chemotherapy, or other hormone therapy.

> Surgery to remove the testicles (orchiectomy) is a form of ADT and is an option for both M0 and M1 castration-naïve prostate cancer.

> ADT might be used alone or with chemotherapy, radiation therapy, steroids, or other hormone therapies.

> Observation is the preferred option for M0 castration-naïve prostate cancer.

> During treatment you will have regular physical exams, PSA tests, and bone scans (if needed).

> If a test shows that your cancer may be progressing, then the next treatment will be based on if there are any metastases.

8
Castration-resistant prostate cancer

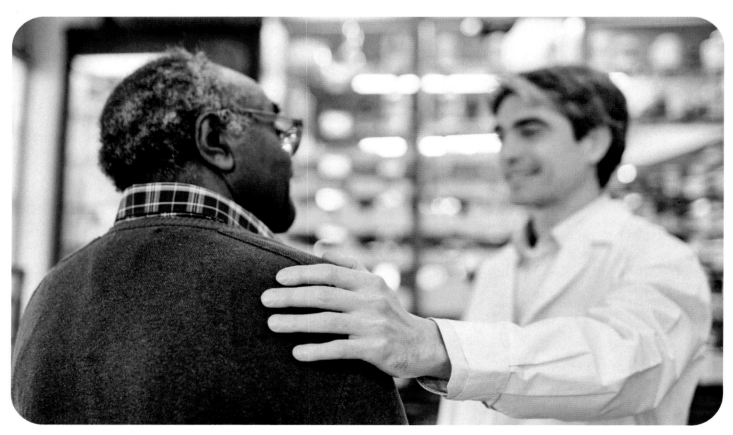

Many early-stage prostate cancers need high levels of testosterone to grow, but castration-resistant prostate cancer (CRPC) does not. Treatment is based on whether or not there are metastases. If there are metastases, treatment is based on the type of metastasis.

Overview

When prostate cancer progresses despite a testosterone castrate level of less than 50 ng/dL, it is called castration-resistant prostate cancer (CRPC). This means that prostate cancer has continued to grow even though testosterone levels are very low. Many early-stage prostate cancers need testosterone to grow, but castration-resistant prostate cancer does not.

Most men with advanced prostate cancer will stop responding to androgen deprivation therapy (ADT). As a result, another hormone therapy might be added to ADT. This is called secondary hormone therapy. As another option, ADT might be added to chemotherapy.

Treatment options are based on if there are:

> No metastases (M0) - If there are no metastases, it is written as M0 CRPC.

> Metastases (M1) and the type of metastases - If there are metastases, it is written as M1 CRPC.

Even though cancer has returned during ADT, it is important to keep taking this therapy. To treat CRPC, testosterone levels need to stay at castrate levels (less than 50 ng/dL). You might stay on your current treatment or your doctor might switch the type of hormone therapy.

Imaging tests might be needed to look for signs of distant metastases.

M0 CRPC

M0 CRPC is castration-resistant prostate cancer without signs of distant metastases. See Guide 10.

Treatment
You will continue to have imaging tests to watch for distant metastases and blood tests to monitor PSA levels. In addition, you will stay on ADT to keep testosterone levels at less than 50 ng/dL. The goal of treatment is to delay the spread of prostate cancer and limit the side effects of treatment.

PSA doubling time (PSADT) will be measured. PSADT is the time it takes for the PSA level to double. Treatment options will be based on PSADT.

PSADT of more than 10 months

If it takes more than 10 months for your PSA to double, then the options are observation (preferred) or another hormone therapy might be added.

PSADT of 10 months or less

If it takes 10 months or less for your PSA to double, then these are your hormone therapy options:

- ➢ Apalutamide (preferred)
- ➢ Darolutamide (preferred)
- ➢ Enzalutamide (preferred)
- ➢ Other hormone therapy

If your PSA level increases with any of the above treatments, then the next steps will be based on whether or not there are metastases.

No metastases (M0)

If there are no metastases, then your doctor will change or keep your current hormone treatment and continue monitoring your cancer. Your doctor will look for signs that your cancer might be getting worse. If your cancer is not getting worse, it may be a sign that the current treatment is keeping your cancer stable.

Metastases (M1)

The following workup will be done to confirm metastases:

- ➢ Bone imaging
- ➢ Chest CT
- ➢ CT of abdomen and pelvis or MRI of abdomen and pelvis
- ➢ Consider PET/CT or PET/MRI

Guide 10
Treatment options: M0 CRPC

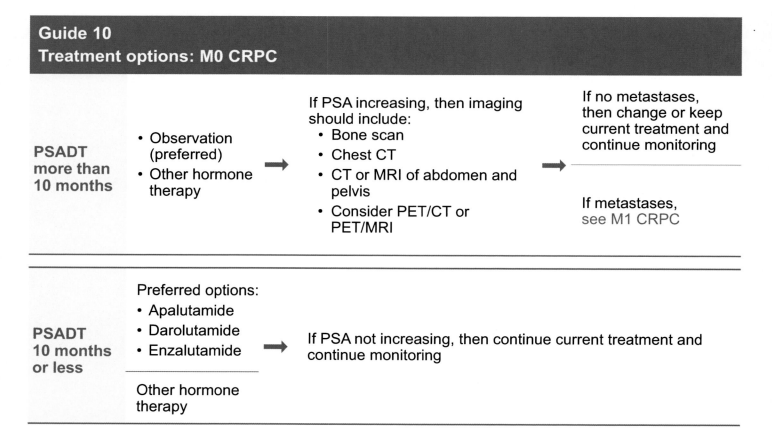

| PSADT more than 10 months | • Observation (preferred)
 • Other hormone therapy | ➡ | If PSA increasing, then imaging should include:
 • Bone scan
 • Chest CT
 • CT or MRI of abdomen and pelvis
 • Consider PET/CT or PET/MRI | ➡ | If no metastases, then change or keep current treatment and continue monitoring

 If metastases, see M1 CRPC |
| PSADT 10 months or less | Preferred options:
 • Apalutamide
 • Darolutamide
 • Enzalutamide
 ——
 Other hormone therapy | ➡ | If PSA not increasing, then continue current treatment and continue monitoring | | |

M1 CRPC

There are different types of metastases:

> Bone

> Lymph and soft tissue

> Visceral (organ)

Low-volume and high-volume are terms used to describe metastases.

> **Low-volume metastatic (M1) disease** includes lymph node metastases and/or 3 or fewer bone metastases.

> **High-volume metastatic (M1) disease** includes visceral metastases and/or 4 or more bone metastases with 1 or more bone metastasis outside the spine or pelvis.

The next section describes treatment options for castration-resistant prostate cancer with metastases (M1 CRPC). These options are based on whether the cancer is or isn't found in the internal (visceral) organs.

M1 CRPC treatment is based on the type of metastases. Bone metastases is cancer that has spread to bones, but not internal (visceral) organs. Visceral metastases are found in the liver, lung, adrenal gland, peritoneum, or brain. The peritoneum lines the abdominal wall and covers most of the organs in the abdomen. Lymph nodes and soft tissues like muscle or blood vessels are not considered visceral.

Testing
Visceral metastases will be biopsied. If not done before, your tumor will be tested for MSI-H or dMMR, germline, and other mutations. Imaging tests will be done to confirm bone metastases.

Small cell or neuroendocrine prostate cancer
If tests find small cell or neuroendocrine prostate cancer, treatment options are chemotherapy and best supportive care.

Chemotherapy options include:

> Cisplatin with etoposide

> Carboplatin with etoposide

> Docetaxel with carboplatin

Treatment overview
You will continue androgen deprivation therapy (ADT) to maintain castrate levels of less than 50 ng/dL.

Treatment for M1 CRPC should include best supportive care. Best supportive care is not cancer treatment. It is treatment to improve quality of life and relieve discomfort.

Options for bone metastases include:

- Bone-targeted therapy (denosumab preferred)
- Palliative radiation therapy for painful bone metastases

First-line treatment

The first-line systemic therapy options for M1 CRPC are listed in Guide 11.

The preferred options are:

- Abiraterone
- Docetaxel
- Enzalutamide
- Sipuleucel-T

It is possible to try all treatment options listed. Best supportive care is always an option.

Radium-223

Radium-223 is an option for metastases that occur mostly in the bones and not in the internal (visceral) organs.

Sipuleucel-T

Sipuleucel-T is an immunotherapy created from your own immune cells. It is used to treat metastatic CRPC where the metastases are in the bone and not in soft tissue, lymph nodes, or visceral organs.

For treatments other than sipuleucel-T, a drop in PSA levels or improvement in imaging tests occurs if treatment is working. This doesn't usually happen right away with sipuleucel-T. Don't be discouraged if your test results don't improve.

Guide 111
First-line therapy options: M1 CRPC

Preferred options:
- Abiraterone
- Docetaxel
- Enzalutamide
- Sipuleucel-T

Radium-223 for bone metastases

Mitoxantrone for pain relief in those with visceral metastases who cannot tolerate other therapies

---

Fine-particle abiraterone

Other hormone therapy

Second-line treatment

The next or second-line therapy is based on whether the first therapy was:

➢ Enzalutamide or abiraterone

➢ Docetaxel

If you were treated with a systemic therapy, then you will try a different therapy than before. It is possible to try all treatment options listed. Best supportive care is always an option. See Guide 12.

Guide 12 Second-line options: M1 CRPC		
Options after enzalutamide or abiraterone	Preferred	• Docetaxel • Sipuleucel-T
	Useful	• Olaparib for HRRm • Pembrolizumab for MSI-H or dMMR • Radium-223 for bone metastases • Rucaparib for *BRCA* mutation
	Other, if not taken before	• Abiraterone • Cabazitaxel • Enzalutamide • Fine-particle abiraterone • Other hormone therapy
Options after docetaxel	Preferred	• Abiraterone • Cabazitaxel • Enzalutamide
	Useful	• Mitoxantrone for pain relief in those with visceral metastases who cannot tolerate other therapies • Olaparib for HRRm • Pembrolizumab for MSI-H or dMMR • Radium-223 for bone metastases • Rucaparib for *BRCA* mutation
	Other, if not taken before	• Consider docetaxel rechallenge • Fine-particle abiraterone • Sipuleucel-T • Other hormone therapy

When M1 CRPC progresses

If castration-resistant prostate cancer progresses, your doctor will try a different therapy than before. It is possible to try all treatment options listed. Options are based on the type of metastasis and tumor mutations. Best supportive care is always an option.

> If docetaxel fails, your doctor may want to try docetaxel again. This is called docetaxel rechallenge.

> Everyone with CRPC should receive best supportive care.

> Talk with your doctor about what you want from treatment. You can always decide not to continue with systemic therapy.

For treatment options, see Guide 13.

Guide 13 Treatment options: M1 CRPC disease progression	
Preferred	One from below if not taken before: • Abiraterone • Cabazitaxel • Docetaxel rechallenge • Enzalutamide
Useful in some cases	• Olaparib for HRRm • Pembrolizumab for MSI-H or dMMR • Mitoxantrone for pain relief in those with visceral metastases who cannot tolerate other therapies • Radium-223 for bone metastases • Rucaparib for *BRCA* mutation
Other, if not taken before	• Fine-particle abiraterone • Other hormone therapy

Review

> Advanced disease is often first treated with androgen deprivation therapy (ADT).

> Castration-resistant prostate cancer (CRPC) is prostate cancer that grows despite very low testosterone levels. It can be metastatic (M1 CRPC) or non-metastatic (M0 CRPC).

> In castration-resistant prostate cancer, if testosterone suppression is not enough to control the cancer, other systemic therapies are needed. ADT continues.

> The goal of treatment for M0 CRPC is to delay the spread of prostate cancer and limit the side effects of treatment.

> Treatment for M1 CRPC is based on whether there are visceral (internal organ) metastases.

> Radium-233 is used for those with bone metastases.

> Sipuleucel-T is used to treat metastatic CRPC where the metastases are in the bone and not in soft tissue, lymph nodes, or visceral organs.

> Everyone with CRPC should receive best supportive care.

9
Making treatment decisions

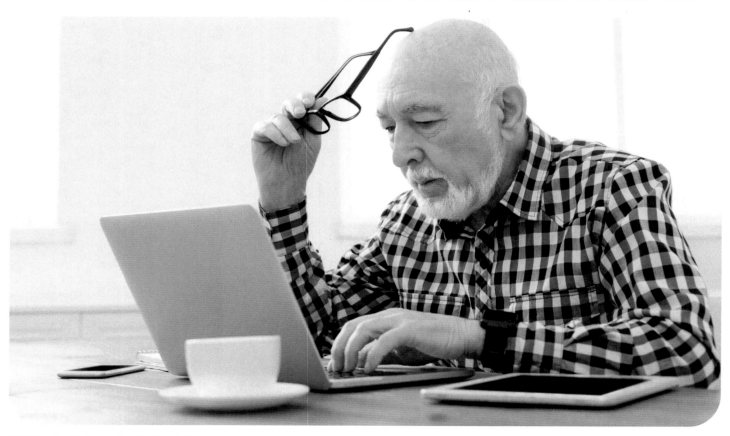

It's important to be comfortable with the cancer treatment you choose. This choice starts with having an open and honest conversation with your doctors.

It's your choice

In shared decision-making, you and your doctors share information, discuss the options, and agree on a treatment plan. It starts with an open and honest conversation between you and your doctor.

Treatment decisions are very personal. What is important to you may not be important to someone else.

Some things that may play a role in your decision-making:

> What you want and how that might differ from what others want

> Your religious and spiritual beliefs

> Your feelings about certain treatments like surgery or chemotherapy

> Your feelings about pain or side effects such as nausea and vomiting

> Cost of treatment, travel to treatment centers, and time away from work

> Quality of life and length of life

> How active you are and the activities that are important to you

Think about what you want from treatment. Discuss openly the risks and benefits of specific treatments and procedures. Weigh options and share concerns with your doctor. If you take the time to build a relationship with your doctor, it

will help you feel supported when considering options and making treatment decisions.

Second opinion

It is normal to want to start treatment as soon as possible. While cancer can't be ignored, there is time to have another doctor review your test results and suggest a treatment plan. This is called getting a second opinion, and it's a normal part of cancer care. Even doctors get second opinions!

Things you can do to prepare:

> Check with your insurance company about its rules on second opinions. There may be out-of-pocket costs to see doctors who are not part of your insurance plan.

> Make plans to have copies of all your records sent to the doctor you will see for your second opinion.

Support groups

Many people diagnosed with cancer find support groups to be helpful. Support groups often include people at different stages of treatment. Some people may be newly diagnosed, while others may be finished with treatment. If your hospital or community doesn't have support groups for people with cancer, check out the websites listed in this book.

Questions to ask your doctors

Possible questions to ask your doctors are listed on the following pages. Feel free to use these questions or come up with your own. Be clear about your goals for treatment and find out what to expect from treatment.

Questions to ask about testing and staging

1. What tests will I have?

2. When will I have a biopsy? Will I have more than one? What are the risks?

3. Will I have any genetic tests?

4. How soon will I know the results and who will explain them to me?

5. Who will talk with me about the next steps? When?

6. What will you do to make me comfortable during testing?

7. Would you give me a copy of the pathology report and other test results?

8. What is the cancer stage? What does this stage mean in terms of survival?

9. What is the grade of the cancer? Does this grade mean the cancer will grow and spread fast?

10. Can the cancer be cured? If not, how well can treatment stop the cancer from growing?

Questions to ask about treatment

1. What are my treatment choices? What are the benefits and risks?

2. Which treatment do you recommend and why?

3. How do my age, health, and other factors affect my options?

4. How long do I have to decide about treatment?

5. When will I start treatment? How long will treatment take?

6. How much will the treatment cost? How much will my insurance pay for?

7. What are the chances my cancer will return? How will it be treated if it returns?

8. I would like a second opinion. Is there someone you can recommend?

9. Which treatment will give me the best quality of life?

10. What in particular should be avoided or taken with caution while receiving treatment?

Questions to ask your doctors about surgery

1. What kind of surgery will I have?

2. What will be removed during surgery?

3. How long will it take me to recover from surgery?

4. How much pain will I be in? What will be done to manage my pain?

5. How will surgery affect my bladder? How long will I need the catheter?

6. What will you do to help with the discomfort of the catheter?

7. How will surgery affect my ability to get and maintain an erection?

8. What are my risks for long-term urinary issues?

9. What other side effects can I expect from surgery?

10. What treatment will I have before, during, or after surgery?

Questions to ask your doctors about radiation therapy

1. What type of radiation therapy will I have?

2. Will you be targeting the prostate alone, or will you also treat the lymph nodes?

3. Will you use hormone therapy with radiation? If so, for how long?

4. How many treatment sessions will I require? Can you do a shorter course of radiation?

5. Do you offer brachytherapy here? If not, can you refer me to someone who does?

6. How does radiation therapy differ from surgery in terms of cure?

7. How will radiation affect my bladder?

8. How will radiation affect my bowels?

9. How will radiation affect my sexual function?

10. What other side effects can I expect from radiation?

Questions to ask your doctors about side effects

1. What are the side effects of treatment?

2. What are my chances of experiencing urinary retention, urinary incontinence, bowel problems, or erectile dysfunction from prostate cancer or its treatment?

3. How long will these side effects last?

4. What can I do to lessen or prevent side effects?

5. What medicines can I take to prevent or relieve side effects?

6. What can I do to help with pain and other side effects? What will you do?

7. Will you stop treatment or change treatment if I have side effects? What do you look for?

8. What side effects should I watch for? When should I call? Can I text?

9. What side effects are life-long or irreversible after completing treatment?

10. What medicines may worsen the side effects of treatment?

Questions to ask your doctors about clinical trials

1. What clinical trials are available for my type and stage of prostate cancer?

2. What are the treatments used in the clinical trial?

3. What does the treatment do?

4. Has the treatment been used before? Has it been used for other types of cancer?

5. What are the risks and benefits of this treatment?

6. What side effects should I expect? How will the side effects be controlled?

7. How long will I be on the clinical trial?

8. Will I be able to get other treatment if this doesn't work?

9. How will you know the treatment is working?

10. Will the clinical trial cost me anything? If so, how much?

Websites

American Cancer Society
cancer.org/cancer/prostatecancer/index

California Prostate Cancer Coalition (CPCC)
prostatecalif.org

Malecare Cancer Support
malecare.org
cancergraph.com

National Alliance of State Prostate Cancer Coalitions (NASPCC)
naspcc.org

National Coalition for Cancer Survivorship
Canceradvocacy.org/toolbox

National Prostate Cancer Awareness Foundation (PCaAware)
pcaaware.org

Nomograms
nomograms.mskcc.org/Prostate/index.aspx

Prostate Cancer Foundation
pcf.org

Prostate Conditions Education Council (PCEC)
prostateconditions.org

Prostate Health Education Network (PHEN)
prostatehealthed.org

Urology Care Foundation
urologyhealth.org

Us TOO International Prostate Cancer Education and Support Network
ustoo.org/Home

Veterans Prostate Cancer Awareness
vetsprostate.org

ZERO - The End of Prostate Cancer
zerocancer.org

Words to know

androgen deprivation therapy (ADT)
A treatment that removes the testes or stops them from making testosterone. Can be achieved through surgery or drugs.

anti-androgen
A drug that stops the action of the hormone testosterone.

best supportive care
Treatment to improve quality of life and relieve discomfort.

bilateral orchiectomy
An operation that removes both testicles.

biopsy
A procedure that removes fluid or tissue samples to be tested for a disease.

brachytherapy
A treatment with radiation from an object placed near or in the tumor. Also called internal radiation.

castration
Surgery that removes the testicles or drugs that suppress the function of the testicles in order to keep testosterone levels low or close to zero.

castration-naive prostate cancer
A worsening of prostate cancer when not on androgen deprivation therapy (ADT).

castration-resistant prostate cancer (CRPC)
A worsening of prostate cancer despite treatment that lowered testosterone.

combined androgen blockade (CAB)
A cancer treatment that stops the making and action of testosterone.

computed tomography (CT)
A test that uses x-rays from many angles to make a picture of the insides of the body.

cryotherapy
A treatment that kills cancer cells by freezing them. Also called cryoablation.

digital rectal exam
A study of the prostate by feeling it through the wall of the rectum.

dual energy x-ray absorptiometry (DEXA)
A test that uses small amounts of radiation to make a picture of bones. Also called bone densitometry.

erectile dysfunction
A lack of blood flow into the penis that limits getting or staying hard.

external beam radiation therapy (EBRT)
A cancer treatment with radiation received from a machine outside the body.

flare
An increase in testosterone after starting treatment to reduce its level.

Gleason grade
A rating of how much prostate cancer cells look like normal cells. A score from 1 (best) to 5 (worst) made by a pathologist based on the ability of prostate cells to form glands. The primary grade is the most common pattern, and the secondary grade is the second most common pattern. The two grades are summed to give a Gleason score.

high dose-rate (HDR) brachytherapy
Treatment with radioactive objects that are removed at the end of the treatment session.

high-intensity focused ultrasound (HIFU)
Treatment using high-intensity sound waves that make heat to kill the cancer cells.

hormone therapy
A cancer treatment that stops the making or action of hormones. Also called endocrine therapy when used for women's cancer. Also called androgen deprivation therapy when used for men's cancers.

image-guided radiation therapy (IGRT)
A treatment with radiation that is aimed at tumors using imaging tests during treatment.

intensity-modulated radiation therapy (IMRT)
Treatment with radiation that uses small beams of different strengths.

intermittent treatment
Alternating periods of time on and off treatment.

life expectancy
The number of years a person is likely to live.

low dose-rate (LDR) brachytherapy
Treatment with radioactive objects that are placed in the tumor and left to decay.

luteinizing hormone-releasing hormone (LHRH) agonist
A drug that acts in the brain to stop the testicles from making testosterone.

luteinizing hormone-releasing hormone (LHRH) antagonist
A drug that acts in the brain to stop the testicles from making testosterone.

magnetic resonance imaging (MRI)
A test that uses radio waves and powerful magnets to make pictures of the insides of the body.

metastasis
The spread of cancer from the first tumor to a new site.

multiparametric magnetic resonance imaging (mpMRI)
A test that makes pictures that show many features of body tissue.

nerve-sparing radical prostatectomy
An operation that removes the prostate and one or neither cavernous nerve bundle.

nomogram
A graphic tool that uses health information to predict an outcome.

observation
A period of testing for changes in cancer status while not receiving treatment.

orchiectomy
An operation that removes one or both testicles.

pelvic lymph node dissection (PLND)
An operation that removes lymph nodes between the hip bones.

perineum
The body region in men between the scrotum and anus.

persistent cancer
Cancer that is not fully treated.

positron emission tomography (PET)
A test that uses radioactive material to see the shape and function of body parts.

prostate-specific antigen (PSA)
A protein mostly made by the prostate. Measured in nanograms per milliliter of PSA.

prostate-specific antigen density (PSAD)
The level of PSA—a prostate-made protein—in relation to the size of the prostate.

prostate-specific antigen doubling time (PSADT)
The time during which the level of PSA—a prostate-made protein—doubles.

prostate-specific antigen (PSA) velocity
How much the level of PSA—a prostate-made protein—changes over time.

radical perineal prostatectomy
An operation that removes the prostate through one cut made between the scrotum and anus.

radical retropubic prostatectomy
An operation that removes the prostate through one large cut made below the belly button.

radiopharmaceutical
A drug that contains a radioactive substance.

recurrence
The return of cancer after a disease-free period.

seminal vesicle
One of two male glands that makes fluid used by sperm for energy.

supportive care
Health care that includes symptom relief but not cancer treatment. Also called palliative care.

surgical margin
The normal-looking tissue around a tumor that was removed during an operation.

testosterone
A hormone that helps the sexual organs in men to work.

three-dimensional conformal radiation therapy (3D-CRT)
A treatment with radiation that uses beams matched to the shape of the tumor.

transrectal ultrasound (TRUS)
A test that sends sound waves through the rectum to make pictures of the prostate.

ultrasound (US)
A test that uses sound waves to take pictures of the inside of the body.

urethra
A tube-shaped structure that carries urine from the bladder to outside the body; it also expels semen in men.

urinary incontinence
A health condition in which the release of urine can't be controlled.

urinary retention
A health condition in which urine can't be released from the bladder.

visceral disease
The spread of cancer from the first tumor to the organs within the belly.

NCCN Contributors

This patient guide is based on the NCCN Clinical Practice Guidelines in Oncology (NCCN Guidelines®) for Prostate Cancer. It was adapted, reviewed, and published with help from the following people:

Dorothy A. Shead, MS
Director, Patient Information Operations

Laura J. Hanisch, PsyD
Medical Writer/Patient Information Specialist

Erin Vidic, MA
Medical Writer

Rachael Clarke
Senior Medical Copyeditor

Tanya Fischer, MEd, MSLIS
Medical Writer

Stephanie Rovito, MPH, CHES®
Medical Writer

Kim Williams
Creative Services Manager

Susan Kidney
Graphic Design Specialist

The NCCN Clinical Practice Guidelines in Oncology (NCCN Guidelines®) for Prostate Cancer, Version 2.2020 were developed by the following NCCN Panel Members:

Edward Schaeffer, MD, PhD/Chair
Robert H. Lurie Comprehensive Cancer Center of Northwestern University

*Sandy Srinivas, MD/Vice Chair
Stanford Cancer Institute

Emmanuel S. Antonarakis, MD
The Sidney Kimmel Comprehensive Cancer Center at Johns Hopkins

Andrew J. Armstrong, MD
Duke Cancer Institute

Justin Bekelman, MD
Abramson Cancer Center at the University of Pennsylvania

*Heather Cheng, MD, PhD
Fred Hutchinson Cancer Research Center/ Seattle Cancer Care Alliance

Anthony Victor D'Amico, MD, PhD
Dana-Farber/Brigham and Women's Cancer Center | Massachusetts General Hospital Cancer Center

Brian J. Davis, MD, PhD
Mayo Clinic Cancer Center

Tanya Dorff, MD
City of Hope National Medical Center

*Jame A. Eastman, MD
Memorial Sloan Kettering Cancer Center

*Thomas A. Farrington
Patient Advocate
Prostate Health Education Network (PHEN)

Xin Gao, MD
Dana-Farber/Brigham and Women's Cancer Center | Massachusetts General Hospital Cancer Center

Celestia S. Higano, MD, FACP
Fred Hutchinson Cancer Research Center/ Seattle Cancer Care Alliance

Eric Mark Horwitz, MD
Fox Chase Cancer Center

Joseph E. Ippolito, MD, PhD
Siteman Cancer Center at Barnes-Jewish Hospital and Washington University School of Medicine

Christopher J. Kane, MD
UC San Diego Moores Cancer Center

Michael Kuettel, MD, MBA, PhD
Roswell Park Cancer Institute

Joshua M. Lang, MD
University of Wisconsin Carbone Cancer Center

Jesse McKenney, MD
Case Comprehensive Cancer Center/ University Hospitals Seidman Cancer Center and Cleveland Clinic Taussig Cancer Institute

George Netto, MD
O'Neal Comprehensive Cancer Center at UAB

David F. Penson, MD, MPH
Vanderbilt-Ingram Cancer Center

Julio M. Pow-Sang, MD
Moffitt Cancer Center

Sylvia Richey, MD
St. Jude Children's Research Hospital/ University of Tennessee Health Science Center

Mack Roach III, MD
UCSF Helen Diller Family Comprehensive Cancer Center

*Stan Rosenfeld
Patient Advocate
University of California San Francisco
Patient Services Committee Chair

Ahmad Shabsigh, MD
The Ohio State University Comprehensive Cancer Center - James Cancer Hospital and Solove Research Institute

Daniel Spratt, MD
University of Michigan Rogel Cancer Center

*Benjamin A. Teply, MD
Fred & Pamela Buffett Cancer Center

Jonathan Tward, MD, PhD
Huntsman Cancer Institute at the University of Utah

NCCN Staff

Deborah Freedman-Cass, PhD
Manager, Licensed Clinical Content

Dorothy A. Shead, MS
Director, Patient Information Operations

* Reviewed this patient guide.
For disclosures, visit www.nccn.org/about/disclosure.aspx.

NCCN Cancer Centers

Abramson Cancer Center
at the University of Pennsylvania
Philadelphia, Pennsylvania
800.789.7366 • pennmedicine.org/cancer

Fred & Pamela Buffett Cancer Center
Omaha, Nebraska
402.559.5600 • unmc.edu/cancercenter

Case Comprehensive Cancer Center/
University Hospitals Seidman Cancer
Center and Cleveland Clinic Taussig
Cancer Institute
Cleveland, Ohio
800.641.2422 • UH Seidman Cancer Center
uhhospitals.org/services/cancer-services
866.223.8100 • CC Taussig Cancer Institute
my.clevelandclinic.org/departments/cancer
216.844.8797 • Case CCC
case.edu/cancer

City of Hope National Medical Center
Los Angeles, California
800.826.4673 • cityofhope.org

Dana-Farber/Brigham and
Women's Cancer Center
Boston, Massachusetts
617.732.5500
youhaveus.org

Massachusetts General Hospital
Cancer Center
617.726.5130
massgeneral.org/cancer-center

Duke Cancer Institute
Durham, North Carolina
888.275.3853 • dukecancerinstitute.org

Fox Chase Cancer Center
Philadelphia, Pennsylvania
888.369.2427 • foxchase.org

Huntsman Cancer Institute
at the University of Utah
Salt Lake City, Utah
800.824.2073
huntsmancancer.org

Fred Hutchinson Cancer
Research Center/Seattle
Cancer Care Alliance
Seattle, Washington
206.606.7222 • seattlecca.org
206.667.5000 • fredhutch.org

The Sidney Kimmel Comprehensive
Cancer Center at Johns Hopkins
Baltimore, Maryland
410.955.8964
www.hopkinskimmelcancercenter.org

Robert H. Lurie Comprehensive
Cancer Center of Northwestern
University
Chicago, Illinois
866.587.4322 • cancer.northwestern.edu

Mayo Clinic Cancer Center
Phoenix/Scottsdale, Arizona
Jacksonville, Florida
Rochester, Minnesota
480.301.8000 • Arizona
904.953.0853 • Florida
507.538.3270 • Minnesota
mayoclinic.org/cancercenter

Memorial Sloan Kettering
Cancer Center
New York, New York
800.525.2225 • mskcc.org

Moffitt Cancer Center
Tampa, Florida
888.663.3488 • moffitt.org

The Ohio State University
Comprehensive Cancer Center -
James Cancer Hospital and
Solove Research Institute
Columbus, Ohio
800.293.5066 • cancer.osu.edu

O'Neal Comprehensive
Cancer Center at UAB
Birmingham, Alabama
800.822.0933 • uab.edu/onealcancercenter

Roswell Park Comprehensive
Cancer Center
Buffalo, New York
877.275.7724 • roswellpark.org

Siteman Cancer Center at Barnes-
Jewish Hospital and Washington
University School of Medicine
St. Louis, Missouri
800.600.3606 • siteman.wustl.edu

St. Jude Children's Research Hospital
The University of Tennessee
Health Science Center
Memphis, Tennessee
866.278.5833 • stjude.org
901.448.5500 • uthsc.edu

Stanford Cancer Institute
Stanford, California
877.668.7535 • cancer.stanford.edu

UC San Diego Moores Cancer Center
La Jolla, California
858.822.6100• cancer.ucsd.edu

UCLA Jonsson
Comprehensive Cancer Center
Los Angeles, California
310.825.5268 • cancer.ucla.edu

UCSF Helen Diller Family
Comprehensive Cancer Center
San Francisco, California
800.689.8273 • cancer.ucsf.edu

University of Colorado Cancer Center
Aurora, Colorado
720.848.0300 • coloradocancercenter.org

University of Michigan
Rogel Cancer Center
Ann Arbor, Michigan
800.865.1125 • rogelcancercenter.org

The University of Texas
MD Anderson Cancer Center
Houston, Texas
844.269.5922 • mdanderson.org

University of Wisconsin
Carbone Cancer Center
Madison, Wisconsin
608.265.1700 • uwhealth.org/cancer

UT Southwestern Simmons
Comprehensive Cancer Center
Dallas, Texas
214.648.3111 • utsouthwestern.edu/simmons

Vanderbilt-Ingram Cancer Center
Nashville, Tennessee
877.936.8422 • vicc.org

Yale Cancer Center/
Smilow Cancer Hospital
New Haven, Connecticut
855.4.SMILOW • yalecancercenter.org

Notes

Index

Made in the USA
Middletown, DE
21 April 2021